An Ethnopharmacologica
of Plants Used by Abagusii Traditional
Medical Practitioners

William Nyang'ate Obiero Gisesa

A substantial amount of content in this book was first published as a thesis submitted for partial fulfillment for the award of degree of Doctor of Philosophy in the Department of Botany, School of Pure and Applied Sciences, Kenyatta University in March 2004.

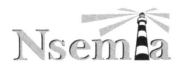

First Edition: September 2024

Published by: Nsemia Inc. Publishers (www.nsemia.com) Oakville, Ontario, Canada

Cover Concept by: Author
Cover Illustration by: Robert Maina Kambo
Cover Design by: Linda Kiboma
Layout Design: Bethsheba Nyabuto

Note for Librarians:

A cataloguing record for this book is available from the Kenya National Library Services.

ISBN: 978-9914-760-07-1

Dedication

To my parents, Kwamboka and Mang'enya who first stressed the importance of education to me.

To my wife, Bochere who has been patient during the period of study.

To my children Kerubo, Mangenya, Nyambega, Morangi and Nyakina.

To my brothers, sisters and their families for their encouragement during the period of study.

To all the people of the world who love nature and would like to go back to nature and are interested in the conservation of biodiversity.

Acknowledgements

I wish to express my sincere gratitude to Prof. Leonard E. Newton and Prof. Sumesh. C. Chhabra for their guidance, invaluable suggestions, sound advice and patience during this project and later in the preparation of this report.

I am also indebted to the entire staff members of the Departments of Botany and Chemistry, School of Pure and Applied Sciences of Kenyatta University for their much-needed help throughout the period of study. I wish to thank Mr. Richard K. Okeyo, Mr. Joseph M. Ogeto, Mr. Omete, Finance Department, Kenyatta University and Sergeant David Omwenga Ong'ayo of Kahawa Garrison, for their moral and financial support during the period of study.

I appreciate the work of the team at Nsemia Inc. Publishers for the diligent efforts they put into getting this publication done. This will make the book reach a wide audience beyond the research and academic communities.

Abstract

An ethno-medical survey of plants used by Abagusii Traditional Medical Practitioners was carried out and 166 plant species representing 138 genera and 62 families were botanically identified. Antimicrobial and phytochemical screening of 20 plants selected from the survey, and reputed to be widely used in the treatment of infectious diseases, was carried out.

The various plant parts (roots, stems, leaves and flowers) of the medicinal plants were Sohxlet extracted with three solvents in order of "increasing polarity (ether, methanol and water). The solvent with the most active extracts (methanol) was used for subsequent extractions of the rest of the plants.

The extracts were screened for bioactivity using the disc diffusion method. Using the same method representative organisms were screened to represent a broad spectrum of micro-organisms including specific clinical isolates from Kenyatta National Hospital.

Tests were performed using the selected plant extracts to find out how effective individual extracts were against specific human pathogens. The phytochemical screening was done by the use of successive and selective extractions with solvents of different polarities (ether, methanol and water). The screening covered mainly nitrogenous compounds, acetogenins, polyketides, isoprenoids and carbohydrates.

In the antimicrobial screening, it was found that most of the plant extracts inhibited the growth of the 7 bacterial species, the fungus and the majority of the 13 pathogenic micro-organisms that they were tested against.

In the phytochemical screening 12 plants (60%) gave a positive reaction for alkaloids, 14 plants (70%) tested positive for tannins, 12 plants (60%) tested positive for flavonoids, 17 plants (85%) tested positive for coumarins, 9 plants (45%)

tested positive for polyketides (emodin), 7 plants (35%) showed the presence of anthocyanins, 7 plants (3 5%) tested positive for anthracene glycosides and 6 plants (30%) showed the presence of fatty acids, 17 plants (85%) showed the presence of steroids/triterpenoids, 13 plants (65%) tested positive for saponins, 17 plants (85%) tested positive for volatile oils and 10 plants (50%) showed the presence of carotenoids, 9 plants (45%) showed the presence of polyuronoids, 11 plants (55%) tested positive for polyoses while 2 plants (10%) showed a positive reaction to starch and 18 plants (90%) tested positive for reducing compounds.

The results show that the local flora has a diversity of plant species with potential medicinal value. The results also confirm that there is credence to many uses which herbalists put in certain plants and their use in traditional medicine and that the plants used by Abagusii Traditional Medical Practitioners are effective against pathogenic micro-organisms. The results supported the hypothesis that the plants used by the Abagusii Traditional Medical Practitioners have compounds of curative value and therefore they play an important role in the basic health care of these people.

Table of Contents

LIST OF TABLES

LIST OF FIGURES

FOREWORD

Before colonialism and the advent of Western religion and medical practices, many African communities, Abagusii included, had developed advanced ways of survival which included knowledge of how to treat various illnesses. Like most indigenous communities across the world, Abagusii not only practised their craft, which they continually improved but also passed the knowledge down generations through elaborate apprenticeship and oral tales. At the centre of managing diseases were plants whose various parts (leaves, roots, bark or a combination thereof) could be used for managing disease. The Abagusii community, which lives in South Western Kenya (straddling the counties of Nyamira and Kisii) had other medical practices, like surgery for head injuries, that were well advanced for their time.

Colonialism, Western Christian religion and Western medical practices came into Kenya in the late 1800s and made a foray into Gusii early in the 1900s. The triple assault on traditional ways of life substantially disrupted the transmission and continuity of many traditional practices. This 'new order' shunned time-tested ways of managing diseases. It was common for these foreigners to label the practices as primitive, evil and unchristian. Indigenous treatment of diseases was further impacted as more and more people converted to the new religion and others acquired a Western education. As such a lot of knowledge was lost as fewer and fewer remained practising the old ways.

Despite this blow, traditional medical treatment survived the assault likely because it was proven and offered results. It is often practised side by side with contemporary ways of treating disease. It is common to see Christians and Western-educated elites turn to traditional healers for medications alongside hospital-prescribed treatments. To a large extent, this affirms the merit of traditional medical practices in the modern world. Indeed, during the COVID-19 pandemic, many traditional

1

healers were reported to have successfully managed cases associated with the virus.

William Gisesa's work examines (using modern scientific methods) the authenticity of the assertions of traditional medicine practitioners. Using a sample of plants used by traditional healers, Dr. Gisesa examined these in a laboratory environment to establish the authenticity of those claims and the efficacy of treatments using the plants.

As results show, the plants in the sample are effective in dealing with the ailment-causing microorganisms (as asserted by the practitioners) when tested in a laboratory environment. It is a major validation of the practitioners' claims about the plants and the diseases they cure. These plants and treatment methods proffered by the healers offer a sound foundation for new medications for the treatment of respective illnesses. Indeed, combined with modern scientific methods for drug formulation and treatment, the potential for plant-based medications is unlimited. Organizations like the Kenya Medical Research Institute (KEMRI) need to take a more prominent lead in this respect.

This work explored only a small number of plants with positive outcomes. Many other plants that were not tested could also hold substantial potential as did those tested. More work by others is required to explore this angle to increase the range of plants and the treatments they could be used for. As the author writes, more efforts and resources need to be directed into these efforts.

The efforts should consider three other issues. The first one is to do an exhaustive recording of the assertions made by traditional healers, i.e. the roaster of plants, the diseases that can be treated using the plants and the manner of administering the cure.

The issue is the conservation of the plants to ensure that they can continue to benefit mankind. The loss of forest cover and the adverse effects of climate change threaten global biodiversity in general. Efforts must be directed at conserving these even as the world explores further ways of extracting value from the plants.

The third aspect relates to the value of this indigenous community knowledge and how that value could be derived for the benefit of the respective communities. Governments should put in mechanisms (laws, policies, processes, treaties, etc.) that would recognize such knowledge as community intellectual property. This way, communities can negotiate with interested parties to ensure they gain from the knowledge even as that knowledge is used for global benefits. Governments, especially in Africa, should exercise this responsibility as a matter of urgency. Done properly, indigenous communities like Abagusii could reap big from such.

On the whole, the work highlights the need for an enforceable policy framework through which such knowledge can come for mainstream use.

Matunda Nyanchama, PhD
Nsemia Inc. Publishers
April 2024

Chapter One

Introduction

1 Uses of Plants

Human beings have always had to rely on plants for their food, shelter, ornamentals, industrial purposes fodder, and other necessities including their medicines, Traditional medicine, based on plants, originally the only healing system known to humans, has never entirely disappeared.

Plants have served as the basis of sophisticated traditional medicine systems for thousands of years in countries such as China and India. These plant-based medicine systems continue to play an essential role in health care in these and many other countries of the world. It has been estimated by the World Health Organization (WHO) that about 80% of the inhabitants of the world especially in developing countries, rely mainly on traditional medicine and medicinal plants for their primary health care (Sofowora, 1982). Plant products also play an important role in the healthcare systems of the remaining 20% of the population who mainly reside in developed countries.

The lore accumulated for millennia by traditional medicine has developed into the modern discipline of ethnopharmacology, the critical study of traditional plant medicines, which has only recently come into its own.

1.2 Development of Traditional Medicine

Traditional medical practice is as old as human history and comprises the beliefs and practices that have been in existence before the development of modern scientific medicine. The knowledge that certain plants possess medicinal value and have been used as a source of drugs by mankind for the treatment of diseases is not new. Historical records also show that some plants were used mainly in the preparation of crude medicaments that were administered to produce relief from numerous ailments suffered by human beings and their livestock (Solecki, 1975).

Early man has put a number of theories forward to explain the acquisition of the knowledge of herbalism. One such theory is that early man deliberately selected specific plant materials for the treatment of his ailments since man has the ability to rationalize rather than rely on instinct as animals do. The choice was certainly not based on a knowledge of the plant constituents. It has also been proposed that knowledge of medicinal plants was gained by accident although this theory has been refuted by a number of traditional medical practitioners who claim that information on such plants was communicated to them by their ancestors in various ways (Akpata, 1979; Lambo, 1979).

However, early man could have gained valuable knowledge concerning the medicinal value of plants through careful observations of animal behaviour. For example, cats and dogs have been known to cure their stomach upsets by eating sharp grasses, while sheep look for *Achillea mellifolium* L. (Compositae). A wild boar suffering from *Hyocyamus niger* L. (Solanaceae) poisoning uses the fresh roots of Carlina *acaulis* L. (Compositae). Mice store heaps of the first days of winter, starving bears look for the flavourful *Allium ursinum* L. (Liliaceae). Ants plant *Thymus vulgaris* L, (Labiatae) all over their habitations to keep fit. If chamois injure themselves, they roll in *Plantago lanceolata* L. (Plantaginaceae). Swallows take the juice of *Chelidonium majus* L. (Papaveraceae) to open the eyes of their young ones and jackdaws keep their nests free of fleas by using tomato leaves. Lizards suffering from snakebite find a cure in *Matricaria chamomilla* L. (Compositae) (Thomson, 1978). Chimpanzees have been noticed to use certain plants when they have particular ailments (Wrangharn, 1975; Rodriguez et al., 1985; Wrangham and Goodhall, 1989).

According to some traditional practitioners (Akpata, 1979; Ogunyemi, 1979), another possibility is that knowledge of traditional cures came from Wizards and Witches. It is believed that some witches, whether living or dead, attend village markets in strange forms: goats, sheep or birds. If someone very shrewd or gifted, such as a traditional practitioner, detects their presence in this disguise the practitioner is promised some useful herbal cures in return for not exposing the witch. The same reward would be offered if a real-life witch was caught in the process of performing an evil act. Hunters, especially in African countries, have been reported as the original custodians of herbal recipes. Such knowledge could have been acquired when, for example, a hunter gist an elephant. If the elephant ran away, chewed leaves from a specific plant and did not die, it is believed the hunter noted the plant as a possible antidote for wounds or for relieving pain.

Traditional practitioners also claim that when in a trance, it is possible to be taught about the properties of plants by the spirit of an ancestor who practiced herbalism. Such a spirit is said to sometimes assume various forms e.g. a large lizard, or a human being with one leg and one arm, using a walking stick. If one encounters such a creature in the dead of night, it can be a useful source of original information on herbal cures (Makhubu, 1978). However,' early man gained his knowledge of the curative powers of plants, one must assume that he was able to recognize the plant since the detailed floras available today were non-existent then.

This inherited, intuitive knowledge of which plant is the right remedy for a given ailment is one of the fascinating aspects of nature and it is not surprising that through trial and error, man learned how to use nature's healing powers for himself. This accumulated knowledge about plants and their medicinal uses was usually passed down from generation to generation verbally. It was customary to pass on this cumulative knowledge to the first son, but occasionally to a trustworthy person (Chhabra et al., 1981).

1.3 World Health Organization (WHO) Policy on Traditional Medicine and Medicinal Plants Research

The fact that some higher plant species have medicinal value cannot be over-emphasized. This fact has been recognized by the WHO, whose Health Assembly has passed several solutions in response to a resurgence of interest in the study and use of traditional medicines and medicinal plants in primary health care and recognition of the importance of medicinal plants to the primary health care systems of many developing countries.

The WHO in its coordinating role has established a working group on traditional medicine in Geneva. Regional directorates of WHO also have some assignments which vary with the overall interest generated in a particular region. The WHO Traditional Medicine Programme has the following as its objectives:

1. To foster a realistic approach to traditional medicine to promote and further contribute to healthcare;

2. To explore the merits of traditional medicine in the light of modern science to maximize useful and effective practices and discourage harmful ones; and

3. To promote the integration of proven valuable knowledge and skills in traditional medicine with Western medicine.

Many international organizations such as WHO, WSCO, UNIDO and AU, which are active in the field of traditional medicine and medicinal plants have made many resolutions on this subject for implementation by member states.

Most of these resolutions recognize the fact that many drugs used in modern medicine can be produced from medicinal plants available in developing countries. They recommend that priority in the production of drugs derived from medicinal plants should be given to drugs that are well-accepted and Widely used throughout the world. Other recommendations center on the recognition of the role of traditional medical practitioners in health care in developing countries, especially in rural populations, which constitute 80-90% of the population in some countries. They urge the developing countries to accord official recognition to those practitioners and have them retrained. Another set of recommendations centres on the education of some members of the modern health teams, as well as medical students, still undergoing training, and urges the inclusion of traditional healing methods on their syllabi (WHO, 1976 -1979; UNIDO, 1978; OAU/STRC, 1979).

The WHO has recommended that there is a need to make an inventory of medicinal plants for each country and that such plants should be analyzed scientifically to determine their efficacy and safety for use by humans and that methods for the safe and effective use of medicinal plants be documented for various levels of health workers. Surprisingly, it was only a few decades ago when the world body formulated this policy despite centuries of use of medicinal plants by human beings.

In reviewing the present status of research into medicinal plants and traditional medicine in Africa, certain important international conferences held on this theme must be mentioned as such conferences have been attended by many African scientists including Anglophone and Francophone ones and the proceedings are an excellent source of detailed information on this topic in Africa. Two of these conferences are the First (OAU)— Inter-African Symposium on Traditional Pharmacopoeia and African Medicinal Plants held in Dakar in 1968 and the Third (OAU) Inter-African Symposium on Traditional Pharmacopoeia and African Medicinal Plants held in Abidjan in 1979.

Before the first OAU symposium in Dakar on medicinal plants, research in this field was uncoordinated and was not particularly application-oriented. Chemists were more interested in isolating and characterizing organic compounds from plants than in discovering whether such compounds had a biological activity or not. Indeed, the plant that was being extracted need not have any therapeutic activity. Although such work provided interesting structural elucidation work for chemists, it had no application for health care. At about this time also, Kerharo and Adams (1974) were listing the medicinal plants of Senegal.

The two workers concluded that with such information work could be started on the investigation of Senegalese medicinal plants, their application to health care and their industrial exploitation. By that time similar work was being carried out in other countries (Brenan, 1949; Dalziel, 1956; Oliver, 1959; Watt & Breyer-Brandwijk, 1962).

This approach changed after the OAU symposium in 1968, probably because, as part of its recommendations, that international meeting decided that collaborative research, centred on finding scientific evidence for the claims of traditional herbal medicine was essential. The executive secretariat of the Organization of African Unity's Scientific, Technical and Research Commission (OAU/STRC) announced also that it was ready to finance centers or groups of research workers working towards such an objective. Both of these factors were very important to the goal of application-oriented research, which marked the next phase.

To provide evidence for the therapeutic efficacy of medicinal plants, multidisciplinary types of research involving pharmacognosists, chemists, pharmacognosists and botanists were necessary. By 1979 most countries in Africa had at least one group of research workers studying the medicinal plants of that country. Most of these groups had multidisciplinary staff attempting the isolation of bioactive agents from plants by monitoring the purification steps by bioassay. Documentation of traditional medical recipes was also initiated in many countries since such recipes were only available orally. Most of these research groups either employed traditional healers as consultants or used them as advisers. Much of the research published in the period between the first symposium and subsequent ones on African medicinal plants up to now reflects this trend of activity along the lines set by the OAU in 1968. This is evidenced by publications made by African scientists in reputable scientific journals in the field of medicinal plants research.

Recently the African Union (AU, 2001) has declared this decade (2001-2010), the decade of African Traditional Medicine, and the World Health Organization African Region (WHO, 2001) has developed guidelines and protocols relating to policy, legal frameworks, research and development methodologies on the promotion of traditional medicine and medicinal plants research in Africa for member states to adopt for use in their national strategic plans and programs.

1.4 The Kenya Government's Policy on Traditional Medicine and Medicinal Plants Research

The government of Kenya's policy on traditional medicine and medicinal plants research is very clear as spelt out in the Kenya Government Development Plan (1989-1993). The Development Plan says the following on the role of traditional medicine: Although for a long time, the role of traditional medicine and its potential contribution to health has been viewed with skepticism, a large proportion of the people of Kenya still depend on it for their cure. One reason for the continued skepticism lies in the lack of information on its effectiveness, drug quality and safety. During the plan period, the Government will encourage the formation of professional associations for traditional medicine practitioners. Such associations will facilitate the gathering of the necessary information for use. development and appropriate adaptation of traditional diagnostic, therapeutic and rehabilitative control technologies that will become part and parcel of formal medical research and the Primary Health Care Programme (PHCP)".

Kokwaro (1991) has reported that about 85% of the Kenyan population, both rural and urban, depends on traditional medicines for their primary health care. However, because of the opposition to the development of traditional medicine from such quarters as conventional medicine, Christianity, modern education, colonialism and the quackery and mysticism surrounding traditional medicine, the Kenya government has a policy of encouraging the formation of professional associations for traditional medical practitioners. Such associations will be charged with the responsibility of gathering information on traditional medicine, plants of medicinal value and any relevant information on traditional medical practices from every ethnic group in the country. In this way, it is hoped that a database will be established that will contain all available information for each plant of medicinal value and its medicinal uses in the various ethnic communities. This information will be used to develop appropriate traditional diagnostic, therapeutic and rehabilitative control technologies that will become part and parcel of formal medical research and the Primary Health Care Programme (PHCP). Such a policy aims to provide a database that will be used in setting up an educational and research programme on traditional medicine and medicinal plants. It is also hoped that through such a policy traditional medicine Will be evaluated scientifically to give information on its effectiveness, drug quality, and safety and to provide a direction for future traditional medical applications and research on medicinal plants

The National Drug Policy (NDP, 1993), being the guidelines adopted nationally offers a clear description of the approach by which pharmaceuticals and pharmaceutical services in the country will be managed. The major goal of the NDP is to use available resources to develop pharmaceutical services that will meet the requirements of all Kenyans in the prevention, diagnosis and treatment of diseases using efficacious, high-quality, safe and cost-effective pharmaceutical products including natural products.

The NDP covers a wide range of activities including traditional medicine, which was given a whole chapter, with the following highlights:

1. Survey of the use of traditional medicines in Kenya;
2. Studying relevant experiences in other countries;
3. Creation of an understanding of the symbiosis of traditional medicine and modern healthcare systems;
4. Development of registration criteria for Traditional Medicine Practitioners;

5. Registration of herbalists at the District level;

6. Development of a national herbal pharmacopoeia;

7. Carrying out studies on toxicity, efficacy and quality of popular cost-effective medicinal plant products to incorporate their use in the health care system; and

8. Carrying out studies on the cultivation of relevant medicinal plants and finally the promotion of selected plants and minerals for use by households, community health workers and other health Workers.

The Ministry of Science and Technology was created and charged with the responsibility of coordinating and facilitating scientific innovations in the country. More specifically the Kenya Medical Research Institute (KEMRI) was charged with the responsibility of evaluating the efficacy of these medicinal plants.

1.5 Area of Study

The area of study encompassed two districts namely Nyamira and Central Kisii Districts comprising of five and six administrative divisions respectfully (Figures 1 a, 1 b, 1 c, and 1 d). The main people living in these two districts are a small Bantu-speaking ethnic group called Abagusii. They speak one common language called Ekegusii.

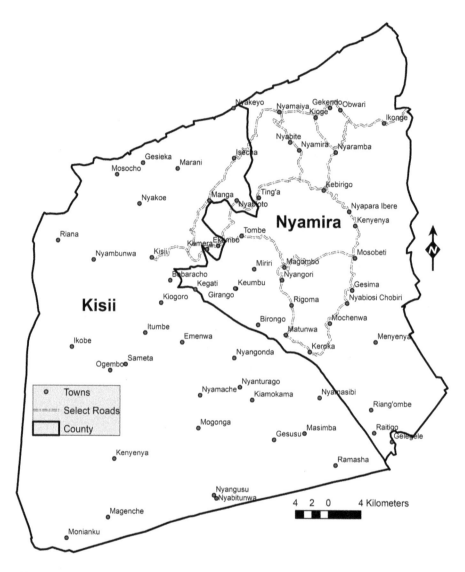

Figure 1: Map of Kisii and Nyamira Counties where the Ethnopharmacology Research took place.

Map Credit: Kefa Otiso

1.6 Ethnographic Information on the Abagusii

Gusiiland, the area in which Nyamira and Kisii Central Districts lie is located in the Nyanza Province of Kenya. it is a cool, fertile highland region with green gently sloping hills with many steep ridges and escarpments. Running between the green hills are swampy streams and rivers. A large expanse of the land is devoid of indigenous trees, removed by increasing population pressure on the scarce available land. Nowadays dark green groves of Australian black wattle, scattered eucalyptus and cypress trees occasionally interrupt the patchwork of crudely terraced fields and pastures.

The Abagusii are among the Bantu-speaking majority of subequatorial Africa, but their entry into the highlands more than two centuries ago isolated them from other Kenyan Bantu people. The Abagusii recognize a common ancestor, Mogusii, who is thought to be the founder of the society and the person after whom it was named. According to oral literature, Mogusii advanced to Nyanza but on reaching the Kisumu area, one group, the Maragoli retreated towards Maseno, another group moved to Subaland and the Abagusii moved and settled on the Gusii highlands, their current residence. Their immediate neighbours are communities of unrelated language families. The Nilotic-speaking Luo to the north, west and southwest, the Nilotic Kipsigis to the east and the Nilotic Masai to the southeast.

In 1907, Gusiiland came under British administration and became part of the South Nyanza District (then known as South Kavirondo) along with the adjacent Luo areas. The Europeans introduced Christianity and then a cash crop economy by encouraging the cultivation of such crops as pyrethrum, tea, black wattle trees for the extraction of tannins for the tanning industry, etc.

This led to the loss of biodiversity, including medicinal plants and indigenous ethno-medical knowledge.

1.7 The Concept of The Causation of Disease Among the Abagusii

Various cultures hold different concepts of diseases and their causation. Most Kenyans hold concepts of disease causation that are characterized by two features: biological basis and all-embracing. The Abagusii are not different either. They believe that humans sustained malfunction due to old age, invasion by organisms such as worms and injuries sustained in accidents. Injurious elements entering the human body system through food, skin and weather changes can also be causes of disease.

The Abagusii also consider man as an integral and extra material entity. They therefore believe that disease can be caused by man due to psychological causes i.e. when his will is not in harmony with the laws of nature. The diseased body is said to be sometimes affected by a diseased state of mind e.g. some people may tend to believe that they are sick they are not sick (hypochondriacs).

The Abagusii also believe that disease can be due to astral influences. They believe that radiations from cosmic agents e.g. the sun, moon and stars have an influence on human beings either for good or for evil. The moon is said to influence the functioning of the brain and it is believed that stammers stammer more in the absence of the moon i.e. during periods of darkness.

Another cause of the disease is thought to be from the spiritual world. Evil thoughts, evil desires and machinations by enemies (i.e. by external influences) including soul projection or evil telepathic messages are all grouped under spiritually caused diseases. Witchcraft is also another cause of disease. Essentially witchcraft is a belief that the spirits of human beings can be sent to go and hurt other persons in body, mind and estate. It is also believed that witches and wizards have psychic powers, which they use to send their spirits to hurt other people.

The other cause of disease comes from esoteric causes. These are diseases originating from the soul, or those caused by the deeds of an individual in his former life (before reincarnation).

The Abagusii believe that diseases can arise from the displeasure of ancestral spirits, and breach the effect of dishonoured oaths. The second group of diseases is generally classified as complicated and serious and therefore their treatment does not only involve material substances like medicinal plants but sometimes includes resources drawn from the immaterial world.

1.8 Aims of the Study

In line with the Kenya Government's policy on the role of traditional medicine and medicinal plants in society, an ethnomedical survey of medicinal plants was carried out in Kisii and Nyamira districts. The gathering of information on the medicinal plants commonly used by Abagusii traditional medical practitioners was carried out through interviews and questionnaires.

Secondly, plant extracts were tested for anti-microbial activity. Thirdly, some plants of medicinal value and which were widely used in the community to treat infectious diseases were selected for screening for compounds of known medicinal value such as nitrogenous compounds, acetogenins, polyketides, isoprenoids and carbohydrates. Lastly, conclusions were drawn about the therapeutic value of the identified medicinal plants and appropriate methods of conservation and the promotion of their uses towards meeting Kenya's development goals are suggested.

1.9 Justification for the Study

For many years, despite the novel compounds plant extracts had and the complex diseases have treated, traditional medicine has been regarded with skepticism and contempt in Kenya the four enemies of the development of traditional medicine have been Christian colonialism, conventional medicine and modern education.

Various religious sects have been known to denounce the practice of traditional medicine and discourage their followers from getting involved with evil spirits through the use of traditional medicine. The colonialists viewed traditional medicine as a cultural nuisance. Both conventional medicine and modern education regarded traditional medicine practices as primitive. Despite all the above resistances to the development of traditional medicine, the following factors make it justifiable to continue to revive interest in research into traditional medicine and medicinal plants:

1. Plants from the tropics are sometimes used as sources of direct therapeutic agents and as starting points for the elaboration of more complex semi-synthetic compounds;

2. Flora from the tropics can serve as sources of substances that can be used as models for new synthetic compounds;

3. There is undisputed clinical efficacy of several plant-based compounds (Mitscher *et al.,* 1987). After searching for synthetic molecules active against the Human Immuno-Deficiency Virus (HIV), reverse transcriptase inhibitors were made. Investigations into plant extracts produced a wide range of compounds that resulted in non-viral proliferation (Kinghorn & Balandilin, 1993);

4. There is also the belief that plants can provide inexpensive renewable sources of feedstock molecules that can readily be transformed into drugs. This renaissance has also been stimulated by the use of plant extracts in treating chronic disease conditions where conventional medicine has offered no help (Sheehan *et al.,* 1992);

5. There is a need to study which plant species are effective in curing diseases. This is bringing science into traditional medicine;

6. There is also the possibility that hidden amongst the myriad of traditional medicinal plant applications there might be a very powerful drug that could be of commercial benefit thus contributing to the national economy and also helping individuals to improve their standards of living e.g. Aspirin started as a local traditional medicine but it has a profound impact in modern medicine and the economies of many countries;

7. A scientific study could also lead to quality control and the ensuring of the correct dosage to be used;

8. Kenya, like most African countries, has a large population, which uses traditional medicine. There have been various attempts to gather information on traditional medicine. However, these attempts to gather information have only concentrated on the uses of medicinal plants. Therefore, there is a need to test the information given in these publications on a scientific basis. Because this kind of investigation is lengthy and requires sophisticated techniques and equipment only a few plants have been investigated in this way;

9. We owe a great deal to traditional medicine. It is the source of our knowledge of many, if not most, of the medicinal plants. Science can continue to learn and profit from the practices of traditional medical practitioners provided we do not allow this rich source of knowledge to dry up;

10. The Aboriginal cultures still extant in the world today - in remote areas of Africa, Asia, and America and elsewhere — are rapidly disappearing. There is a danger that much of the knowledge and practice of the alleviative properties of plants will vanish with these cultures. It is not too soon to pay serious attention to this popular healing tradition and to review some examples of the pharmacological contributions it has made to the past- and can go on making —to modern medicine and our knowledge of medicinal plants;

11. A continent of rich and varied tropical floras- and the home of man: Africa harbours millions of natives still living in primitive societies, yet ethnobotanical studies of some of these societies are lacking. Some publications on the toxic and medicinal plants of East, South and West Africa suggest that investigations of some of the medicinal plants still used by the natives could lead to medically valuable discoveries (Watt & Breyer-Brandwijk, 1962);

12. In Africa, in general and Kenya in particular, there are very few ethnobotanicals; and

13. There are not many studies that have been undertaken. For instance, no ethnobotanical study has been done on the Abagusii ethnic group. This is also one of the reasons that this study was undertaken.

1.10 Hypothesis

The medicinal plants used by Abagusii traditional medical practitioners have active ingredients that are of curative value and therefore play a key role in the primary care of these people.

1.11 General Objective

To carry out an ethnomedical survey, antimicrobial and phytochemical screening of medicinal plants used by Abagusii Traditional Medical Practitioners.

1.12 Specific Objectives

1 To carry out an ethnomedical survey and gather information on the medicinal uses of plants used by the Abagusii traditional medicinal practitioners through interviews and questionnaires.

2 To identify botanically the medicinal plants used.

3 To give priority to commonly used plants to be used for chemical and biological

4 To screen extracts of the twenty most widely used medicinal plants from the results.

5 To screen twenty of the most widely used plants for classes of compounds of medicinal value such as nitrogenous compounds, acetogenins, polyketides, isoprenoids, carbohydrates, etc.

To conclude the medicinal value of the plants investigated and suggest appropriate methods for their conservation.

Chapter Two

Literature Review

2.1 Uses of Medicinal Plants

Plants have been used as a source of drugs for humans for several thousands of years. More than 200,000 out of the approximately 350,000 or more plant species so far identified in the whole of our planet are in tropical countries in Africa and elsewhere. Among the potential users of these plants, traditional medicine and pharmacopoeia are on top of those who practice them, that is, 80% of the population of the Third World (Sofowara, 1982).

2.2 Why the Interest in Ethnopharmacology?

African medicinal plants have long provided important sources of healing drugs to local populations. The information obtained from ethnomedicine is now being put on a scientific basis and it is therefore very important to investigate the chemical, biological, pharmacological and phytochemical aspects of different preparations from different vegetable sources. This type of research requires an interdisciplinary approach in which botanists, ethnobotanists, phytochemists, biologists and pharmacologists work together to unravel the mysteries.

There is a certain urgency associated with this work since plant habitats are being changed or destroyed daily and it is essential to study as much of the disappearing plant materials as soon as possible before the opportunities are lost. Another factor is that with the decreasing number of traditional healers, the accumulation of their valuable knowledge is progressively diminishing. This source of priceless data also needs to be exploited before it is too late.

The third factor is that modern medicine owes a lot to ethnomedicine. Some of the better-known and widely used plant medicines used today such as quinine from the genus *Cinchona* *morphine* from the opium poppy and many others started simply as herbal medicines (Sofawora, 1982).

2.3 Major Drugs of Plant Origin That Are Widely Used Today

Malaria is a protozoan disease that is endemic in Africa and many parts of the world. It is a major killer, but many drugs have proved useful in the treatment of this disease. One of these is quinine, a drug derived from the bark of various species of the South American trees of the genus *Cinchona* (Trease & Evans, 1978). Indians had used this plant from the earliest times and introduced it to Catholic missionaries in the 17th century. The drug, which consists of four alkaloids, is extracted from the dried bark by dissolving it in alcohol. Nowadays, synthetic drugs such as atabrine are used to treat malaria, but quinine is still employed on a considerable scale. The drug is used to prevent muscle cramps and in small quantities, as a flavouring for 'tonic' drinks.

Since the dawn of history, people have known that a powerful drug could be obtained from the seed vessels of a common poppy plant, *Papaver somniferum*. Its use was recorded by the ancient Egyptians, the Greeks and the Romans. In modern medicine, opium is used mainly as a source of the drug morphine, which is extracted by complex chemical processes. Morphine is mainly used to deaden pain arising from an accident or disease. It also controls coughing in respiratory diseases and induces a feeling of euphoria or well-being. No satisfactory substitute has yet been found for it. Moreover, it is the only narcotic that relieves pain in reasonably safe doses (Le Strange, 1977; Trease, & Evans, 1978; Taylor, 1975).

The belladonna plant, *Atropa belladonna*, often called the deadly nightshade, grows wild in woods and waste places in Europe and is cultivated in Holland to provide the leaves and roots that yield certain patent drugs. Chemists extract from the dried powdered leaves and also from the roots, two drugs called atropine and hyoscine that relax certain muscles and dry various glands. It has been claimed that there are over 50 medicinal uses of atropine ranging from the treatment of asthma to the relief of indigestion. It can be used to increase the heart and lower blood pressure. It is frequently given before an operation to reduce salvation and prevent sickness (Trease & Evans, 1978; Taylor, 1965; Le Strange, 1977).

Pharmacologists were puzzled by how one drug could exert so many diverse actions. it is now realized that atropine prevents the passage of nerve impulses across the neuromuscular joint. Large doses, especially atropine, cause delirium and subsequently send patients into a comma. Atropine also causes the pupil of the eye to dilate (Trease & Evans, 1978; Taylor, 1965; Le Strange, 1977).

Strychnine plants, mainly *Strychnos nux-vomica*, which yield two stimulating drugs, strychnine and brucine are small trees, bushes and climbers of several species. Its main use in modern medicine is in awakening people out of narcotic comas. It also increases the acuteness of certain sensory perceptions (Trease & Evans, 1978).

Cocaine is the only widely used local anesthetic of plant origin though there are several synthetic ones. An injection of a tincture of cocaine has the effect of deadening the responses of nerves in small areas of the body to pain for periods of up to one hour. It is widely used in dentistry. The drug is obtained from the coca tree, Erythroxylon coca. (Taylor, 1965; Le Strange, 197 7; Trease & Evans, 1978).

The foxglove, *Digitalis purpurea*, leaves are ground into a powder and are then used in the treatment of a failing heart (Taylor, 1965; Le Strange, 1977). Digitalis contains several glycosides. These acting together improve the productive work of the heart while slowing the pulse rate. Despite several years of effort, digitalis has never been prepared in the laboratory nor has any synthetic product been found which can completely replace it. Infusions of dried foxglove leaves were used for centuries by simple country folk who knew nothing about its complicated action but were satisfied simply to know that it could relieve the edema, which often accompanied congestive heart failure.

2.4 The Use of Herbal Medicine in Africa

The African continent, like all other continents, has had its uses for medicinal plants. Most of the countries on the continent still depend on traditional medicine for their primary healthcare. For example, lemon grass, *Cymbopogon citratus* DC., which contains citral oil, grows in many parts of Africa (Watt & Breyer-Brandwijk, 1962). In Congo, citral oil is used to treat leprosy and can be applied on the forehead and face to relieve headaches. In Ghana, Liberia, Nigeria, Sierra Leone and Guinea Bissau, it is used to provide antispasmodic relief (Onawunmi et al., 1984).

Achyranthes aspera L. which is found in many parts of East and West Africa is used widely for medicinal purposes (Watt & Breyer-Brandwijk, 1962). *Ageratum conyzoides* L is a common weed that grows in many parts of Africa and is used as a remedy for all sorts of abdominal upsets, for the relief of abdominal pains, as a remedy for fresh wounds and to cure syphilitic sores. In Central Africa, the leaf is used to aid the healing of wounds, especially those caused by burns. In East Africa, the leaves of the plant have been used as a haemostatic and to stop epitasis or any type of bleeding from injury (Kokwaro, 1993).

Acacia nilotica (L) Del. is a typical African plant (Watt & Breyer-Brandwijk, 1962). It grows in South Africa, West Africa, Sudan, Egypt, Ethiopia and Tanzania. The Maasai of Tanzania uses the bark as a nerve stimulant. The Zulus of South Africa use it to loosen a dry cough, while in West Africa the bark is regarded as a tonic and is used internally for diarrhea and dysentery.

Bauhimia reticulate DC., which is found in many parts of both East and West Africa, is widely used for medicinal purposes (Watt & Breyer-Brandwijk, 1962). It is used in Zambia for the treatment of malaria, anthrax and dysentery. In Congo and Guinea, it is used against leprosy while in West Africa, the bark and roots are used as a remedy for coughs, worms and malaria. The roots of a different species, *Bauhinia rufescens* Lam, are used in Niger to cure fevers (Marston & Hostettmarm, 1993).

In Nigeria, a legume, *Tetrapleura tetraptera Taub.*, is used for the treatment of several diseases (Ojowole & Adesina, 1983) including the management of convulsions, leprosy, inflammation and rheumatic pains. It has been established through field trials that it is very potent in the control of schistosomiasis (Hostettmann & Hostettmann, 1989).

Johns et al. (1990) reported that 330 species in 254 genera are used for the treatment of ailments by the Luo in Kenya. Kioy (1989) has reported on the use of *Warburgia ugandensis* for the treatment of diseases such as malaria, coughs and joint pains among some Kenyan ethnic groups. Mensah and Achenbach (1987) have argued, after considering recent research trends, that there is credence to the number of uses which herbalists put in certain plants and their use in modern medicine. Even in modern medicine, the drugs are derived from medicinal plants and then synthesized in chemical factories. One can, therefore, argue that conventional medicine is an extension of herbal medicine.

In some countries, in Africa, despite the lack of concrete studies, researchers express little doubt that plant medicines are still widely used. This is thought to be increasing due to the rising cost of Western drugs and negative experiences with modern drugs and the modern healthcare system (Gbile & Adensia, 1987).

For example, in one Ashante village in Ghana, Amponsah-Agyemang (1980) found that traditional medicine was still of great importance. He found that even though half of the population was Christian and there was no fetish priest in the village, all the villagers that were interviewed regularly employed traditional plant medicines.

2.5 Antimicrobial Compounds from Plants

2.5.1 Antimicrobial Activities of Plant Extracts

It is now clear medicinal plants are active against micro-organisms (Galloway et al., 1991; Irobi, 1992; Encamacion & Gaza, 1991; Irobi & Daramola, 1994; Paulo et al., 1992; Grein & Brantner, 1994).

Chinese herbs such as *Ledebouviella seseloides* Wolff and *Potentilla chinensis* L. have activity against *Staphylococcus aureus* (Chang & But, 1987; Galloway *et al.,* 1991). In British Columbia, several plants used medicinally were screened for antibacterial activity (McCutcheon *et al.,* 1992). Seventy-five percent of these plants had antibacterial activity against methicillin-resistant *Streptococcus aureus* and many of them were active against *Pseudomonas aeruginosa.*

In Guatemala, out of the sixteen medicinal plants used for gastrointestinal disorders and screened for activity, eight (50%) of them inhibited the growth of *Salmonella flaxineri* (Caceras *et al.,* 1993). In North America, *Rhus glabra* L. which is used traditionally by the native Indians for the treatment of bacterial diseases is active against eleven species of bacteria (McCutcheon *et al.,* 1992). The organisms most affected are *P. aeruginosa, Escherichia coli* and *S. aureus.* Plants, such as *Bursera microphylla* A. Gray, *Wislizenia refracta* Engelm var. *palmeri* and *Bacharis glutinosa* Pers. were found to inhibit the growth of *S. aureus* (Encarnacion *et al.,* 1991).

In Pakistan and India, *Mimosa humata* Willd. is active against *Mycobacterium smegmatis* and *E. coli* (Hussein *et al.,* 1979). Another indigenous plant Uvaria narum Wall. which is used traditionally for the treatment of skin and mucosal infections inhibits the growth of *Salmonella typhi, E. coli* and *Klebsiella aerogenes.*

In Africa, *Acalypha wilkesiana* Muell-Arg. which grows widely in Southern Nigeria inhibits the growth of *S. aureus* and *Trichophyton rubrum* (Alade and Irobi, 1993). Another plant in the same region, *Dalbergia melanoxylon* Guill. and Perr., which is used locally for cleaning wounds and for the treatment of gonorrhea is active against *Salmonella typhimurium, Yersinia pestis* and *Klebsiella pneumoniae* (Gundidza and Gaza, 1993). In Tanzania, out of 85 plant extracts examined, 32% had activity against *Salmonella typhi, P. aeruginosa, Shigella dysenterica* and *Klebsiella pneumoniae* (Chhabra *et al.,* 1981). In Kenya *Commiphora rostrate* has been found to exhibit antimicrobial activity against *Aspergillus flaxus, Aspergillus niger* and some *Penicillium* spp (Mcdowell *et al.*, 1988).

2.5.2 Antimicrobial Compounds Identified in Plants

In the United Kingdom and North America, almost 26% of the active components of currently prescribed medicines were first identified in plants (Balandalin *et al.*, 1925). By the middle of the 20th Century, certain groups of compounds such as alkaloids were known to be responsible for the biological activity observed in drug-producing plants (Sheehan *et al.*, 1992). This observation led to the screening of other plants for similar compounds that could be detected by simple chemical tests. Currently, new activities and chemical substances are reported for plants with a long history of traditional medicinal use.

Plant compounds such as artemisinin and forkolin presently being developed as antimicrobial drugs have been mentioned elsewhere (Kinghorn and Balandalin, 1993; Phillipson *et al.*, 1993). Chloroquine, which has been used for several years, is well known (White *et al.*, 1992). Recently other compounds have been isolated with promising potency (Sakanaka *et al.*, 1989; Kubo *et al.*, 1992; Taniguchi and Kubo, 1993).

In the past none of the top 250 pharmaceutical companies in the Western Society did research on plants and their biological effects (Fellows, 1992). Now over half of these companies make efforts toward uncovering new, clinically useful antibiotics in higher plants (Mitscher *et al.*, 1972). Several individual articles have been published in which results of large screening studies are given. The List can be long but the few examples given above serve as an illustration that antibiosis is not uncommon among higher plants. The potential for finding useful chemotherapeutic agents in plants is therefore reasonable.

2.6 Ethnomedical Survey

Traditional societies in Africa and elsewhere have always relied on plants for their food and other necessities, including their medicines (Chhabra *et al.*, 1984). Such societies had devised methods of providing everybody in the community with essential health care through acceptable, affordable and accessible means by the application of indigenous resources such as plants, animals, mineral products and certain other methods. Even today, despite the high advances in modern medicine, people still attach great importance to the traditional system of medicine because it takes into account their socio-cultural backgrounds.

African traditional medicine abounds in medicinal plants and the people, wherever they live, rely on traditional medicine. The Abagusii are no exception. In addition to the herbalists who enjoy great prestige as the real practitioners of traditional medicine, divine healers and witchdoctors also employ medicinal plants that are supposed to have either special spiritual or exorcising powers.

Attempts have been made to gather information on traditional medicine, medicinal plants and the people who use them (Kokwaro, 1993; Watt & Breyer-Brandwijk, 1962; Timberlake, 1986; Tanaka, 1980; Morgan, 1981; Lindsay, 1978; Barrett, 1996). However, only a small number of plants have been identified. Moreover, these publications have not covered all the communities in Kenya, the Abagusii included.

2.7 Antimicrobial Screening

In many studies dealing with the effects of antimicrobial compounds on micro-organisms usually representative micro-organisms from Gram-positive and Gram-negative bacterial and fungal species are used (Tanira *et al.,* 1994; Pomilio *et al.,* 1992; Akunyili *et al.,* 1991). This procedure was also followed in this investigation.

2.8 Phytochemical Screening

Basic phytochemical screening consists of performing simple chemical tests to detect the presence of classes of compounds such as nitrogenous compounds, acetogenins, polyketides, isoprenoids, carbohydrates, etc., that are known to be of medicinal value in a plant extract (Trease & Evans, 1978).

The general composition of an unknown vegetable product may be determined using qualitative chemical analysis by extraction with different solvents of different polarities through successive and selective extractions, thus leading to the separation of the main classes of chemical constituents.

The first step in such a procedure is to select the plant material, dry it and then reduce it to powder. Secondly, the powdered vegetable drug is extracted with a lipophilic solvent e.g. ether (a less polar solvent). Following this, the vegetable product is extracted with ethyl or methyl alcohol (an intermediate polar solvent) and finally with water (a strong polar solvent). Three extractive solutions are thus obtained namely: the ether extract (E), methanol extract (M) and the water extract (W). The ether extract will contain the lipophile chemical constituents and the other two polar solvents, the hydrophile constituents.

2.9 Examples of Potential Uses of Medicinal Plant Extracts

African medicinal plants constitute a rich, but untapped pool of natural products with important potential uses. For example, the biological activities of the alkaloids are remarkable. Distinct fungicidal activities of the alkaloids with relevance to crop protection have been found (Bringmann & Proksch, 1992). Already extracts of *Triphophyllum peltatum* are highly active against important plant-pathogenic bacteria. This fungicidal activity is most likely to give the plant a specific advantage in the humid rain forest. The same protective effect can be expected from a strong antifeedant and growth-inhibiting activity against insects, tested on the polyphagous generalist *Spodoptora littoralis*- a well-established (largely toxin-resistant) herbivore model system (Bringmann *et al.*, 1996).

One of the presently exciting biological properties of the alkaloids is their anti-malarial activity. Approximately a third of the world's population lives in malaria-endemic areas, and more than 2-3 million people die of malaria each year. (Bringmann *et al.*, 1996). Many *Plasmodium* strains, especially P. *falciparum* have become resistant to classical anti-malarial drugs such as chloroquine. Therefore, due to the rapid spread of the disease, the search for new anti-malarial agents is an urgent task. Extracts of some *Ancistrocladus* species used in traditional medicine have been shown to exhibit high vistro activities against P. *falciparum*, and also against chloroquine-resistant strains (Francois *et al.*, 1994). The above anti-malarial and anti-bilharzial activities of the alkaloids are of greatest importance since such tropical diseases take a high toll on lives in the tropical countries where the plants grow. Recently, *Ancistrocladus* alkaloids have become candidates as possible drugs against the immunodeficiency disease AIDS - one great medical and social challenge of our time.

Plants provide some very powerful molluscicidal agents, and therefore, a large amount of effort has been spent over the last few years in the discovery of new molluscicides (Mott, 1987) Alkaloids have been found to have molluscicidal activity against the tropical snail *Biomphalaria glabrata*, the immediate host of the tropical disease bilharziasis (schistosomisis), which is so widespread in Africa. Besides the direct chemotherapy of bilharzia, the patients, another strategy is to kill the snails to disrupt the parasitical cycle. One of the most promising plants for the potential control of schistosomiasis-transmitting snails in Africa, besides *Phytolaca dodecandra* (Phytolaccaceae) is *Swartia madagascariensis* (Leguminosae). Aqueous extracts of the seedpods contain large amounts of saponins with high molluscicidal activity. These saponins have been characterized and field trials with extracts of the fruits have been performed in Tanzania (Hostettman & Hostettmann, 1989).

Plant extracts have also been implicated in wound healing. In plants, gums and related compounds affect wound healing, by acting as protective agents that cover accidental wounds (Ross & Brain, 1977). Plants possess groups of chemical compounds implicated in the primary repair of tissues, which include: polysaccharides and specifically, glycosaminoglycans, and polyuronides (Ikan, 1969), some of which are found as main constituents of mucilages and gums (Ross & Brain 1977; MacGregor & Greenwood, 1980). Some of these compounds, which also possess antibiotic and/or antimicrobial properties, offer a double advantage in wound healing.

Some chemical compounds, which are released by plants after and in response to injury, have been tested on zoological pathogens, some of which may be implicated in causing wounds (Adesanya & Roberts, 1995).

Propolis, a resinous substance found in beehives collected by bees from buds, has been used in the treatment of wounds (Magro-Filho & de Carvalho, 1994) just as honey is used. The future of plant extracts externally in the management of wounds is bright because there is a growing interest in the clinical practice of wound management with the use of chemical component-impregnated dressings (Morris et al., 1994). African traditional medical practitioners have, over the years, also been treating various wounds with traditional medical remedies. Mucilages are used as a soothing application to the mucous membranes (Ellis & Calne, 1977).

In Ghana, *Euphorbia hirta* L. leaves are used in sore and wound healing. It is used in East Africa to treat boils (Sofowora, 1996). *Borreria verticillata* (Rubiaceae) is used in Casamance for the treatment of whitlow boils, by applying a paste obtained by pounding the leaves in a mortar with the extract of *Carapa procera*. The volatile oil it contains is rich in terpenes, phenolics and aromatic polycarboxylic acids. The high boiling components of the volatile oil have shown strong antimicrobial activity against Gram-positive and Gram-negative bacteria (Sofowora, 1996). The chemical compounds with wound-healing activity are not restricted to a particular chemical group. They are, however, mostly proteins, amino acids, terpenes, flavonoids, alkaloids, quinonoids, tannins, steroids, carbohydrates or coumarins. Many triterpene saponins and their aglycones have been reported to possess antiulcerogenic, anti-inflammatory, fibrinolytic, antipyretic, analgesic and anti-edermatous activities. The saponins are reported to act by promoting mucous formation (Hostettmann *et al.,* 1995). This property favours wound healing by preventing wound desiccation as well as furnishing important growth factors.

Reports in the literature (Watt & Breyer-Brandwijk, 1962; Gelfand *et al.,* 1985; Kokwaro, 1993) indicate that traditional healers throughout Africa have confined themselves almost exclusively to the use of the genus *Combretum* and a lesser extent the *Terminalia* in the treatment of a wide range of maladies. In the last two decades, a series of stilbenes and dihydro stilbenes (the combretastatin) with potent cytotoxic activity and acidic triterpenoids and their glycosides with molluscicidal, antifungal, antimicrobial and anti-inflammatory activity have been isolated from species of Combretum (Rogers, 1989 & 1989 b).

The bitter leaf exudates of some Aloe species are commercially important sources of the laxative aloe drug and are also used in the cosmetics industry as additives in shampoos, shaving and skin care creams and in the treatment of skin disorders and in particular as a topical medication for the treatment of burns (Rowe *et al.,* 1941).

The well-known cathartic drug, Cascara bark, is derived from the Asian *Rhamnus purshiana* DC. Bark. The leaves and stems of *Rhamnus prinoides* are indispensable ingredients in the making of traditional fermented beverages in Ethiopia. The fruits are, however, used in the treatment of ringworm infections. The role of *R. prinodes* in the fermentation process has been investigated (Kleyn & Hough, 1971; Sahle & Gashe, 1991) and it is claimed that the plant regulates the microflora responsible for the fermentation process. It has also been reported that the extracts of *Rhamnus. prinoides* be used as a commercial hopping agent for beer (Tessema, 1994). Senna is an important genus, which has yielded important purgative drugs. The biologically active constituents of *Senna* are the hydroxy anthracene glycosides known as *sennosides.*

The fact that plants have invariably been a rich source of new drugs and some anti-drugs in use today (quinine and artemisinine) cannot be doubted. Some of these compounds were either obtained from plants or developed using their chemical structure as templates (Gessler *et al.,* 1994). However, it has been shown that *Plasmodium falciparum*, the most Widespread etiological agent for human malaria is becoming increasingly resistant to standard antimalarial drugs which necessitated a continuous effort to search for new antimalarial drugs. However, over the years, the scientific progress in malaria chemotherapy has been more or less on the effects of already existing drugs than on the development of new ones. The search for new antimalarial drugs has regained importance due to the resurgence of drug-resistant strains in many countries. Malaria chemotherapy and prophylaxis are now targeting drug combinations with the hope of achieving drug potentiation to circumvent or delay resistance (Zucker, 1993; WHO, 2000). In Southeast Asia, the use of first-line drugs with artemisinin derivatives such as artesunate has been shown to increase efficacy, protect drugs against resistance and increase the life span of antimicrobial compounds (TDR, 2000). Reports of resistance to sulfadoxine-pyrimethamine, which is currently used as a first-line drug, are on the increase (WHO, 1998; USN, 2001).

Chhabra et al. (2003) have reported the *in vitro* antiplasmodial activity and chloroquine potentiation effects of fifty-five organic and aqueous extracts of 11 plants used in malaria therapy in Central Kisii District, Kenya. This investigation revealed that the combination of some extracts of these plants with chloroquine against the multi-drug resistant *Falciparum* isolate VI/S produced synergistic effects. They concluded that the plant extracts with low IC 50 values might be used as sources for novel antimicrobial compounds to be used alone or in combination with chloroquine.

The list of the potential uses of medicinal plant extracts in the treatment of various human disease conditions is undoubtedly lengthy and the multiplication of examples would not serve any useful purpose. The medicinal value of some of those plant extracts in primary health care cannot be overemphasized.

Chapter Three

Ethnomedical Survey

3.1 Materials and Methods

An ethno-medical survey was carried out in Nyamira and Central Kisii Districts in Nyanza Province, Kenya (Figures 1 a, and 1 b). Several villages in the study area were visited. For the selection of the villages, the District Officer (DO) in charge of the administrative division (Figures 1 c and 1 d) was contacted. The area DO issued a letter of introduction to the chief. The chief passed on the introductory letter to the assistant chief, who in turn introduced the researcher to the village elder, who knew the place well and also the homes of the traditional medical practitioners. Ten villages were selected from each division. The selection was based on Where the traditional medical practitioners lived. 1100 traditional medical practitioners were interviewed. The information on the ethnomedical practices gathered from the traditional healers was entered into questionnaires (Appendix) and field notebooks.

The healers were quizzed about their knowledge and methods of diagnosis) preparation of herbal potions and the treatment of diseases. The specific plant part(s) used along with the methods of preparation were recorded. This work was done between April and August 1997 during the long rains when there was plenty of vegetation.

The plant specimens were collected and pressed in a plant press and placed in the herbarium to dry at room temperature. Their vernacular names were recorded while in the field. The plants collected were allotted collection numbers G001 to G166. They were then identified using the Kenyatta University Botany Department's Herbarium and the East African Herbarium. For each plant specimen collected, the vernacular name, botanical name and ethnomedical uses(s), method of preparation of the medicinal potion and toxic effects, if any, were documented. Voucher specimens were deposited in the Department of Botany, Kenyatta University.

3.2 Results

One hundred and sixty plant species representing 138 genera and 62 families commonly used by the Abagusii traditional medical practitioners were botanically identified. The results are presented below.

AGARICACEAE

Agaricus campestris L. Ex Fries (G001) (Image on page 182)

Vernacular name: Oboba

Use(s) and preparation: An emetic.

3 cups of a decoction of the dried plant of the common mushroom made in 1 litre of water are drunk and as an emetic

AGAVACEAE

Agave americana L. (exotic) (G002) (Image on page 182)

Vernacular name: Rikonge

Use(s) and preparation: wounds, infectious diseases, digestive disorders, jaundice, hepatitis and edema.

2.3 cups of an infusion made of 50 g of roots or ground leaves per litre of water, sweetened with honey are drunk three times daily as a remedy for edema and the retention of fluids in the body system. For bruises and skin wounds, compresses with the juice or sap of the leaves are applied on the affected skin area.

ALOACEAE

Aloe vera (L.) Burm. f. (Syn Aloe barbadensis Miller) (Exotic) (G003) (Image on page 184)

Vernacular name: Omogaka

Use(s) and preparation: Stomach ulcers and problems; is an appetizer, a laxative and a purgative, proves uterine contractions (oxytoci), increases menstrual flow; treats burn and fungal infections, improves the appearance of scars and cracks in the skin; is a digestive and treats duodenal ulcers

2-3 spoonfuls of aloe juice dissolved in water. Fruit juice or milk is taken three times daily to enhance its effects during the treatment of skin infections e.g. eczema. For burns, compresses are recommended. These are pasted on the affected area for a day. However, they are resoaked in more aloe juice every time till they become dry. At night animal fat is applied because aloe juice dries the skin. In the treatment of skin diseases such as eczema, any type of lotion is applied with aloe juice 2-3 times daily on the affected area. It is recommended that such treatment should be accompanied by some emollient (soothing) oil.

AMARANTHACEAE

Achyranthes aspera L. (G004) (Image on page 182)

Vernacular name: Esarara

Uses(s) and preparation: Syphilis, an emesis and anti-malaria, toothache. and stomach problems

The young stem is chewed until it achieves brush-like ends, dipped in common salt and used as a brush to clean teeth. 10 g of the ash of the burnt ash of the dried whole plant is mixed with 1 glass of water and boiled. 2-3 cups of this decoction are drunk three times daily after every meal as a remedy for stomach problems. 100 g of fresh leaves are macerated and then mixed with flour, and boiled to make a paste which is used as a poultice and applied on boils and abscesses to hasten their maturity so that the pus can be squeezed out of them and herbal treatments are applied to hasten their healing.

ANACARDIACEAE

Mangifera indica L. (exotic) (G005) (Image page 202)

Vernacular name: Riembe

Use(s) and preparation: Ringworm, diarrhea, and insomnia.

10 g of woody tissue is burnt into ash. 1 teaspoonful of the ash is mixed with animal ghee and pasted on an area infected with ringworm. 3-4 cups of an infusion made from 20-30 g of leaves per litre of water and sweetened with honey are drunk daily after every meal as a remedy for diarrhea. 2-3 cups of an infusion of 10 g of leaves in 1 litre of water are drunk when somebody is retiring to bed as a remedy for insomnia.

Rhus vulgaris Meikle (G006) (Image on page 210)

Vernacular name: Obosangora

Use(s) and preparation: Diuresis, wounds, diarrhea; and toothache.

10 g of fresh or cooked fruits are eaten daily by a person suffering from scurvy 2 cups of a decoction made from 20 g of root material in one litre of water are drunk after every meal as a treatment for scurvy. A decoction made from 10 g of ground stem material made in 1 litre of water is mixed with 5 g of common salt and is applied directly on wounds with the help of cotton wool. Young slender stems are chewed until they achieve brush-like ends and are then used to clean teeth.

APOCYNACEAE

Carissa edulis (Forssk.) Bahl. (G007) (Image on page 188)

Vernacular name: Omonyangateti

Use(s) preparation: Gonorrhoea, pelvic pain, backache, indigestion, lower abdominal and chest pains.

3-4 cups of a decoction prepared from 10 g of root material in 1 litre of water and sweetened with a cup of honey are drunk daily as a remedy for indigestion, lower abdominal pains during pregnancy and malaria.

3-4 cups of an infusion made from 20-30 g of root material per litre of Water are drunk daily for the treatment of chest pains.

Rauvolfia caffra Sond. (G008) (Image on page 209)

Vernacular name: Omomure

Use(s) and preparation: Gonorrhoea and other sexually transmitted diseases.

3 cups of a decoction made from 10-15 g of dry powdered root material in 1 litre of water are drunk daily

Tabernaemontana stapfiana Britten (G009) (Image on page 215)

Vernacular name: Omobondo.

Use(s) and preparation: Gonorrhoea and other sexually transmitted diseases.

2-3 cups of a decoction made from 10-15 g of dry powdered root material in 1 litre of water are drunk daily.

ASPLENIACEAE

Dryopteris filix-mas Schott. (G 010) (Image on page 193)

Vernacular name: Eengwe

Use(s) and preparation: Anthelmintic

5 g of the powder of the rhizome and the root are swallowed.

Warning: During the treatment, no alcoholic beverages should be taken. No more than 10 g of the powder should be swallowed because the plant is toxic.

BASELLACEAE

Basella alba L. (G011) (Image on page 185)

Vernacular name: Enderema

Use(s) and preparation: Constipation.

10-20 g of fresh leaves are macerated and strained and the extract mixed with 1 litre of and 3-4 cups are chunk three times daily for constipation.

CACTACEAE

Pachycereus pectin-aboriginum L (exotic). (G012) (Image on page 206)

Vernacular name: Omobimbera ng'umbu

Use(s) and preparation: wound healing

5 g of the leaves are macerated and strained and the extract is used to clean wounds when there is no water around. When the bleeding has stopped a piece of cactus is tied around the wound with a piece of cloth. After 2-3 hours the strip is removed from the wound.

Opuntia ficus- indica (L.) Miller (exotic) (G013) (Image on page 205)

Vernacular name: Omote bwa' amakengo.

Use(s) and preparation: Diarrhea, coughs, lack of urine production and cystitis.

For the treatment of diarrhea, the fruit is carefully rinsed and eaten. For the treatment of a cough, syrup is prepared by slicing the fruit and covering it with brown sugar. This is steeped for twelve hours, strained and drunk hot in spoonfuls for lack of urine production and cystitis.

CAESALPINACEAE

Caesalpinia decapetala (Roth) Alston (exotic) (G014) (Image on page 186)

Vernacular name: Ekenagwa

Use(s) and preparation: Gonorrhoea

3-5 cups of a decoction made from 100 g of root material are drunk daily

Cassia didymobotyra Fresen (Syn *Senna didymobotrya* (Fresen.) Irwin and Barneby) (GO15) (Image on page 188)

Vernacular name: Omobeno.

Use(s) and preparation: Purgative, gonorrhea, backache; appetizer, ringworm, measles, fever and headache.

50 g of ground leaves and 50 g of ground stems are mixed with 1 litre of water. This decoction can also be made with leaves only in a proportion of 100 g of leaves per litre of water. This is then boiled for twenty minutes. 3-4 cups are drunk daily as a remedy for gonorrhea and also given to weaned children to act as an appetizer. 5 g of burnt ash from the whole plant is mixed with one teaspoonful of ghee and pasted on an area infected with ringworm. 200 g of ground root material are boiled in 1 litre of water and the decoction is used as a water bath for the treatment of measles three cups are drunk as are boiled in one litre of water and one cup of the decoction is drunk after every meal as a remedy for malaria fever and headache.

Cassia floribunda Cav. (Syn *Senna septemtrionalis* (Viviani) Irwin & Barneby) (GO16) (Image on page 188)

Vernacular name: Omobeno omwegarori.

Use(s) and preparation: Purgative; gonorrhea, backache, an appetizer, ringworm, measles, stomach problems, fever and headache.

50 g of ground leaves and 50 g of ground stems are mixed with 1 litre of water. This decoction can also be made with leaves only in a proportion of 100 g of leaves per litre of water. This is then boiled for twenty minutes. 3-4 cups are drunk daily as a remedy for gonorrhea and also given to weaned children to act as an appetizer. 5 g of burnt ash from the whole plant is mixed with one teaspoonful of ghee and pasted on an area infected with ringworm. 200 g of ground root material are boiled in 1 litre of water and the decoction is used as a water bath for the treatment of measles and three cups are drunk as a remedy for stomach problems. 50 g of leaves and 50 g of roots are boiled in one litre of water and one cup of the decoction

is drunk after every meal as a remedy for malaria fever and headache.

Cassia occidentalis L. (Syn *Senna occidentalis* (L.) Link.) (G017) (Image on page 188)

Vernacular name: Omote ogotioka

Use(s) and preparation: Fever, snake bite, kidney problems) inflammations, edema, bruises, dysmenorrhea, furuncles, sprains, prostate glands, purgative, and an antispasmodic substance.

For internal use a decoction made from 100 g of the root material per litre of water is boiled until its volume is reduced to a third of the original volume strained and sweetened with honey and 2-3 cups are drunk after each meal as a remedy for painful menstruation. For prostate disorders, a teaspoonful of toasted seeds, ground into a powder, are mixed with 1 cup of water and drunk daily after every meal. For external use, poultices of leaves are used as a remedy for edema, bruises, furuncles and sprains.

CAMPANULACEAE

Lobelia gibberoa Hemsl. (G018) (Image on page 202)

Vernacular name: Omomoa/Etumbato enyegarori

Use(s) and preparation: Stimulant, diaphoretic, skin diseases, chronic rheumatism and gout

2 cups of an infusion of 20-30 g of the powder of the whole plant made in 1 litre of water are drunk as a stimulant and a diaphoretic. A decoction of 100-200 g of flesh leaves in 1 litre of water is used to bathe the whole body of a person with any skin malady, chronic rheumatism or gout.

CANELLACEAE

Warburgia ugandensis Sprague (G019) (Image on page 220)

Vernacular name: Esoko/Omonyakige.

Use(s) and preparation: Chest pains, malaria and toothache.

4 cups of a decoction made from 20-30 g of the roots and bark in 1 litre of water are drunk daily.

CANNABIACEAE
Cannabis sativa L. (exotic) (G020) (Image on page 187)
Vernacular name: Enyasore

Use(s) and preparation: Painkiller

An infusion with a teaspoonful of seeds is made, steeped for 30 minutes and 1-2 cups are drunk.

Warning: It is addictive and therefore its use is not recommended.

CAPPARIDACEAE
Gynandropsis gynandra (L.) Briq. (G021) (Image on page 199)
Vernacular name: Chinsaga

Use(s) and preparation: Dissolves adhesions in the womb and increases the production of milk.

3 cups of a decoction made from 20 g of the roots of the plant in 1 litre of water are drunk to dissolve adhesions in the womb. The soft young tender leaves are cooked and eaten by lactating mothers to improve milk production.

CARICACEAE
Carica papaya L. (exotic) (G022) (Image on page 187)
Vernacular name: Ripaipai

Use(s) and preparation: Ringworm, sterility in women, high blood pressure, venereal diseases, constipation, flu, scorpion stings, skin rashes, upset stomachs and intestinal worm.

1 green fruit is cut and rubbed on an area infected with ringworm. 1 yellow fruit is cut into pieces, boiled in one litre of water and 5 g of common salt is added to the decoction. 3 cups of this decoction are drunk daily as a remedy for

sterility in women. 1 green or yellow fruit is pounded with five oranges and this mixture is boiled in 1 litre of water 3-4 cups of this decoction is drunk daily as a treatment for high blood pressure. 3 cups of an-infusion made from 10 g of the leaves of the male plant per litre of water are drunk daily for the treatment of sexually transmitted diseases, constipation and flu. For scorpion stings a concentrated infusion made from 50 g in 1 litre of water is used to wash an area that has been stung by scorpions, 50 g of yellow or old leaves are boiled in 10 litres of water and allowed to cool then used to bathe children as a remedy for rashes. The raw fruit is cut into pieces and eaten by people, especially old people complaining of an upset stomach when they eat meat, chicken or eggs. 3-4 teaspoonfuls (15-20 ml) of the milky latex that comes out when the green tree trunk is cut are collected and then mixed amount of honey and stirred in a cup of hot water. This is taken with a laxative e.g. castor bean oil. 3 cups of this are drunk daily until the worms are completely expelled.

CHRYSOBALANACEAE

Parinari curatellifolia Benth (G023) (Image on page 206)

Vernacular name: Omoraa

Use(s) and preparation: A haemostatic; epitasis, sore eyes, bowel complaints, stomachache and coughs.

50 g of fresh leaves are macerated and then strained and the extract is used as eye drops. This extract is also mixed with common salt and applied on fresh wounds to stop bleeding and also to hasten the process of healing, 100 g of fresh leaves are boiled in one litre of water, allowed to cool and then sweetened with honey. 1 cup of this decoction is drunk daily after every meal as a cure for stomachache, bowel complaints and coughs.

COMBRETACEAE

Combretum molle G. Don. (G024) (Image on page 190)

Vernacular: Kamukira

Use(s) and preparation: Stomachache and coughs.

100 g of fresh leaves are boiled in one litre of water, allowed to cool and then sweetened with honey. 1 cup of this decoction is drunk after every meal as a cure for stomachache and coughs.

COMMELINACEAE
Commelina benghalensis L. (G025) (Image on page 190)

Vernacular name: Rikongiro

Use(s) and preparation: Fevers

100 g of the leaves are boiled in 1 litre of water and used as a wash.

Pentarrhinum insipidium L. (G026) (Image on page 207)

Vernacular name: Ogoto kw'embeba

Use(s) and preparation: Stomachache

40-50 g of leaves are macerated and dropped in 1 litre of water and strained. 2-3 cups of this infusion are drunk as a remedy for stomach pains.

COMPOSITAE
Ageratum conzyoides L. (G027) (Image on page 183)

Vernacular name: Emete y'amaiso

Use(s) and preparation: A haemostatic, epitasis; sore eyes, bowel complaints

50 g of fresh leaves are macerated and then strained. The resulting extract is used as eye drops. This extract is also mixed with salt and applied to fresh wounds to stop bleeding and also, to hasten healing, 100 g of fresh leaves are boiled in one litre of water, allowed to cool and then sweetened with honey. 1 cup of this honey is drunk after every meal as a cure for stomachache, bowel complaints and coughs.

Bidens grantii (Oliv.) Sherff. (G028) (Image on page 185)

Vernacular name: Rirarang'era

Use(s) and preparation: Stomach troubles

One cup per litre of an infusion of 30 g of leaves of *B. grantii* and 30 g of the leaves of *Ocimum basilicum* per litre of water and sweetened with honey is drunk before every meal.

Bidens pilosa L. (G029) (Image on page 186)

Vernacular name: Ekemogamogia.

Uses and preparation: Wound healing, earache, rheumatism, abdominal troubles, pain diarrhea and colic.

10g of the leaves are macerated, mixed with common salt and pasted on a fresh wound to stop bleeding and hasten its healing. 100 g of the fresh leaves are macerated and mixed with 1 litre of water to make and used as eardrops. 2-3 drops are dropped into an aching ear. Seeds are toasted and ground into fine powder and this powder is rubbed on incisions made on the side of the trunk for the relief of pain. 1000 g of flowers are boiled in 1 litre of Water to make a decoction and one cup of this decoction is drunk three times daily as a remedy for diarrhea. 50 g of the leaves and 50 g of the roots are macerated in 1 litre of water to make an infusion. 1 cup of this infusion is sweetened with 1 cup of honey and drunk three times daily after every meal as a remedy for colic.

Chrysanthemum cineriaefolium (Trev.) Bocc. (exotic). (G 030) (Image on page 188)

Vernacular name: Riuga

Use(s) and preparation: Scabies

A decoction made from 100g of the dried and ground flowers made in 1 litre of water is used to bathe the whole body of a person suffering from scabies.

Cnicus benedictus L. (Syn *Centaura benedicta* L.) (G031) (Image on page 189)

Vernacular name: Rigeria nyagutwa

Use(s) and preparation: Digestive atony, lack of appetite, bloated stomach, vomiting, diabetes, wounds, skin sores and hemorrhoids.

2-3 cups of an infusion or decoction of 20-30 g of fresh or dry leaves per litre of water are drunk daily as a remedy for digestive atony, lack of appetite, bloated stomach and vomiting. If the herbal tea is too sour it is sweetened with some honey or brown sugar. For the cleansing of wounds, and skin sores compresses soaked in a decoction with a handful of leaves, stems and/or flowers per litre of water are applied locally on the affected area, and for hemorrhoids, the same decoction is used in the baths.

Crassocephalum vitellinum (Benth.) S. Moore. (G032) (Image on page 190)

Vernacular name: Entamame

Use(s) and preparation: Wounds; diseased eyes, gonorrhea, suppurations of the skin and improves the quality of milk in a lactating woman.

10 g of flowers are macerated and mixed with l g of common salt and directly applied to a bleeding wound to stop the flow of blood and to hasten the healing process. 50 g of the leaves are pounded and then boiled in 1 litre of water and the decoction is used as eye drops. 1 cup of the same decoction is drunk three times daily after every meal as a remedy for gonorrhea, and suppurations and to improve the quality of milk in a lactating mother.

Dichrocephala integrifolia O. Kuntze (G033) (Image on page 193)

vernacular name: Ekeng'enta mbori

Use(s) and preparation: Thrush.

2 spoonfuls of the ash are stirred in 1 glass of fresh milk and given to the child to drink.

Erlangea marginata L. (G034) (Image on page 194)

Vernacular name: Omonyaiboba

Use(s) and preparation: Sores, fungal infections and skin rashes.

A decoction made of 50-60 g of leaves in one litre of Water is mixed with 10 g of common salt and then applied to the sores. A decoction of 100 g of pounded leaves made in 1 litre of water is used to bathe areas infected with ringworm. A decoction made from 1000 g of fresh leaves in 1 litre of Water is used to bathe the whole body as a treatment for skin rashes.

Galinsoga parviflora Cav. (G035) (Image on page 198)

Vernacular name: Omenta

Use(s) and preparation: Sores.

10 g of the leaves are macerated, mixed with common salt and pasted on a sore

Helianthus annus L. (exotic). (G036) (Image on page 199)

Verncular name: Riuga ri'omogaso

Use(s) and preparation: Bronchial catarrh, respiratory afflictions, diabetes, liver afflictions, certain skin afflictions such as eczema and furuncles

For bronchial and respiratory afllictions-4 cups of an infusion made from 100 g of flowers and the young stems in 1 litre of water are drunk daily whereas in the treatment of diabetes, liver affliction and certain skin afflictions such as eczema and furuncles, oil from the seeds is used.

Leonotis nepetifolia R. Br. (G037) (Image on page 202)

Vernacular name: Risibi

Use(s) and preparation: Stomachache.

10-20 g of the leaves are macerated in 1 litre of water and 3 cups of this infusion are drunk daily for the relief of stomachache.

Psiada arabica Jacq. (G038) (Image on page 209)

Vernacular name: Omosune omonyerere

Use(s) and preparation: Aphrodisiac; vertigo, general pains and malaria.

2-3 cups of a decoction made from 30-40 g of fresh leaves in 1 litre of water are drunk. 3-4 cups of root/leaf decoction made from 100 g of root tissue in 1 litre of water are drunk daily as a remedy for vertigo and as an aphrodisiac. 2-3 cups of root and leaf decoctions are drunk three times a day as a treatment for general abdominal pains. The same decoction is also drunk as a malaria remedy.

Solanecio mannii (Hook. f.) C. Jeffrey (G039) (Image on page 213)

Vernacular name: Omotagara

Use(s) and preparation: Stomachache.

10-20 g of the leaves are macerated in 1 litre of water and 3 cups of this infusion are drunk daily for the relief of stomachache.

Spilanthes mauritiana (A. Rich) DC. (G040) (Image on page 215)

Vernacular name: Ekenyunyunta monwa

Use(s) and preparation: Thrush, diarrhea and excessive bleeding during menstruation. 3-4 cups of an infusion made from 20-40 g of leaves are drunk daily for the treatment of sores in the mouth of young children (thrush). 3-4 cups of a decoction made from 40-50 g of leaves in 1 litre of Water are drunk daily as a remedy for diarrhea and excessive bleeding during menstruation.

Tagetes minuta L. (G041) (Image on page 215)

Vernacular name: Omotiokia

Use(s) and preparation: Wound healing

10 g of fresh leaves are macerated and the macerate is mixed with 1 g of salt and pasted on a fresh wound to stop bleeding

and hasten the healing process. Alternatively, dry leaves are ground into powder, mixed with ghee and pasted on a fresh wound. The wound is then tied with a piece of cloth.

Taraxacum officinale Weber ex. Wiggers (G042) (Image on page 216)

Vernacular name: Etandalioni

Use(s) and preparation: Laxative.

2 cups of a decoction made from 10 g of the dried rhizome and 10 g of the roots in 1 litre of water are drunk three times daily as a remedy for constipation.

Tithonia diversifolia (Hemsl.) Gray (exotic). (G043) (Image on page 217)

Vernacular name: Riuga riroro

Use(s) and preparation: Stomach pains, and dislocated joints.
2-3 cups of an infusion of 30 g of leaves per litre of water are drunk three times daily as a remedy for stomach pains. A handful of leaves warmed over a fire is used for massaging a dislocated organ.

Vernonia auriculifera Hiern. (G044) (Image on page 219)

Vernacular name: Omosabakwa

Use(s) and preparation: A treatment of fever and aching breasts.

4 cups of an infusion of 30-40 g of leaves in 1 litre of water are drunk three times daily as a remedy for fever. 20g of buds macerated are mixed with animal ghee and used to massage aching breasts.

Vernonia amygdalina Del. (G045) (Image on page 219)

Vernacular name: Omonyamosuto (Omorororia)

Use(s) and preparation: Aching breasts.

20g of buds macerated are mixed with animal ghee and used to massage aching breasts.

CONVOLVULACEAE

Ipomoea batatas L. (exotic) (G046). (Image on page 201)

Vernacular: Amanyabwari

Use(s) and preparation: Antihelmintic

20-30 g of leaves are macerated in 1 litre of water and strained. The extract is drunk for the expulsion of hookworms from the gut.

CUCURBITACEAE

Cucumis prophetarum L. (G047) (Image on page 191)

Vernacular name: Omwatekania

Use(s) and preparation: Swollen organs and problems of indigestion.

Leaves are mixed with animal fat and used to massage a swollen organ. 10 g of macerated leaves are mixed with animal fat and used to massage a swollen organ. 1 cup of an infusion made from 20 g of leaves and 20 g of stern tissue is drunk three times daily as a remedy for indigestion.

Cucumis disaceus Spach. (G048) (Image on page 191)

Vernacular name: Obuya

Use(s) and preparation: Fresh wounds, swollen neck glands; an emetic, purgative; and an antidote for poisoning.

5 g of root tissue and 5 g of leaf tissue are macerated, mixed with 5 g of table salt and pasted on fresh wounds to hasten their healing. 10 g of fresh fruit tissue are mashed and dropped into ½ litre of water. Common salt is added and is used to massage swollen neck glands. 20 g of root tissue and 20 g of fruit tissue are pounded together, dropped into 1 litre of boiling water, allowed to cool, and then strained, and 4-5 cups are drunk as a purgative.

Cucurbita maxima L. (Syn *Cucurbita pepo* L.) (G049) (Image on page 191)

Vernacular name: Omwongo

Use(s) and preparation: Antihelmintic

10 g of fresh fruit tissue is cut into pieces and boiled. 1 litre of water and 4-5 cups are drunk as a purgative. 4-5 cups are drunk as an anti-helmitic.

Lagenaria siceraria (Molina) Standley (G050) (Image on page 201)

Vernacular name: Ekerandi

Use(s) and preparation: A purgative.

1000 g of roots and fruit are burnt into ash. 1 spoonful of this ash is stirred in 1 cup of hot water and given to young to act as a purgative.

Mormodica foetida Schumach (G051) (Image on page 204)

Vernacular name: Egwagwa

Use(s) and preparation: Thrush.

100 g of the buds are boiled in 1 litre of water and 3-4 cups of the extract are drunk.

CUPRESSACEAE

Cupressus sempervivens L. (exotic). (G052) (Image on page 191)

Vernacular name: Ebakora/Ekerobo

Use(s) and preparation: Varicose veins, varicose ulceration, hemorrhoids and uterine hemorrhages.

For varicose veins, varicose ulcerations and hemorrhoids, a decoction of 50 g of ground fruits or the same amount of wood in 1 litre of water is boiled for 30 minutes and strained. 1 cup of this decoction is drunk after each meal. 3 cups are drunk daily. For hemorrhoids, a concentrated decoction i.e. 100 g of nuts per litre is used in a bath. Three baths are recommended daily

CRUCIFERAE
Brassica oleraceae L (G053) (Image on page 186)
Use(s) and preparation: Ekabichi nyamato

Use(s) and preparation: Gastro-duodenal ulcers, diabetes, Intestinal worms, wounds, varicose and torpid ulcers, eczema, furuncles and acne.

For gastro-duodenal ulcers, 1 cup of fresh juice is drunk three to four times daily before each meal on an empty stomach. Poultices, prepared with either raw leaves or cooked leaves mixed with bran so that the mixture becomes more compact, are applied directly on an affected skin area for the treatment of infected wounds, varicose veins, torpid ulcers, eczema, furuncles and acne.

CYPERACEAE
Cyperus rotundus L. (G054) (Image on page 192)
Vernacular name: Endwani

Use(s) and preparation: Fevers

The bulb is boiled and eaten for fevers.

DIOSCOREACEAE
Dioscorea minutiflora Engl. (exotic) (G055) (Image on page 193)
Vernacular name: Chinduma

Use(s) and preparation: Measles.

Tubers are boiled or roasted and given to small children to eat to help in expelling intestinal worms.

Warning: They should be soaked in cold water first to dissolve poisonous compounds.

EBENACEAE
Bridelia micrantha (Hochst.) Baill. (G056) (Image on page 186)
Vernacular name: Omotarakanga

Use(s) and preparation: Purgative.

2-3 cups of a root decoction made from 50 g of the roots in 1 litre of water are drunk.

EUPHORBIACEAE

Croton macrostachyus Del. (G058) (Image on page 190)

Vernacular name: Omosocho

Use(s) and preparation: Diarrhea and dysentery.

50 g of the dry leaves are ground into a powder. Two spoonfuls of this powder are stirred in one cup of water and drunk as a remedy for diarrhea and dysentery.

Euphorbia hirta L. (G059) (Image on page 195)

Vernacular name: Obwaranse

Use(s) and preparation: Thrush, diarrhea and dysentery.

10 g of leaves are combined with 10 g of the leaves of *Oxalis latifolia* and 10 g of *Ajuga remota* macerated and strained. 1 cup of this extract is recommended as a remedy for children suffering from a condition in which the mouth becomes bloody red. 50 g of the dry leaves are ground into a powder. Two spoonfuls of this powder are stirred in one cup of water and drunk as a remedy for diarrhea and dysentery.

Euphorbia tirucalli L. (G060) (Image on page 196)

Vernacular name: Ekerachwoki

Use(s) and preparation: wounds, sore throat, stomach complaints, snake bite and sterility in women.

The milky latex is applied on wounds. 2- 10 ml of the latex is mixed with one cup of fresh milk and drunk as a treatment for sore throat and stomach complaints. 4 cups of the decoction made from 20 g of the roots in 1 litre of water are drunk as an emetic and for sterility in women.

Warning: Highly toxic. Take care.

Flueggia virosa (Willd) Voigt. (Syn *Securinega virosa* (Willd.) Baill.) (G062) (Image on page 197)

Vernacular name: Esarara

Use(s) and preparation: Chest pains

4 cups of a decoction made from 40 g of roots in 1 litre of water are drunk daily.

Manihot esculentum Crantz. (G063) (Image on page 203)

Vernacular name: Omwogo

Use(s) and preparation: Snake bites, boils, abscesses, sores, diarrhea, dysentery, flu and marasmus.

10 g of fresh tubers are cut into small pieces and pounded into a paste. A little water (100 ml) is added to the paste and incisions are made on the site of a snakebite and the paste is rubbed on these. Flour from the tuber is made into poultices and used in the treatment of boils sores and abscesses. 4-5 cups of porridge made from the finely ground tubers are drunk as a remedy for diarrhea and dysentery. An infusion made from 100 g of leaves per litre of water is used to bathe the whole body for the treatment of flu and marasmus.

Phyllanthus avalifolius Forssk. (exotic) (G064) (Image on page 208)

Vernacular name: Omonyanaigo

Use(s) and preparation: Healing of the navel.

2-3 cups of a decoction made from 30-40 g of the leaves per litre of water are drunk once a day to hasten the healing of the navel of a newborn baby. At the same time, the decoction is used to bathe the baby for the same purpose.

Ricinus communis L. (exotic) (G065) (Image on page 211)

Vernacular name: Omobono

Use(s) and preparation: Constipation.

One cup of the oil extracted from the seeds is drunk as a laxative or purgative depending on the dosage.

Tragia bethamii L. (G066) (Image on page 217)

Vernacular name: Enyangeni/Enyanduri.

Use(s) and preparation: Healing of the navel.

2-3 cups of a decoction made from 30-40 g of the leaves per litre of water are drunk once a day to hasten the healing of the navel of a newborn baby. At the same time, the decoction is used to bathe the baby for the same purpose.

FLACOURTIACEAE

Dovyalis abyssinica L. (G067) (Image on page 193)

Vernacular name: Omokorogonywa

Use(s) and preparation: gonorrhea, bilharzia, stomachache and fever.

3-4 cups of 20 g of the root decoction made in 1 litre of water boiled with fat is drunk as a treatment for stomachache and fever.

GRAMINEAE

Agropyron repens (L.) Beauvois (G068) (Image on page 182)

Vernacular name: Ekenyambi

Use(s) and preparation: Cystitis and other diseases of the genital tract.

10 g of the dried rhizome are macerated in 1 litre of water and the extract is filtered. 3-4 cups are drunk daily.

Bambusa vulgaris L. (G069) (Image on page 184)

Vernacular name: Emoti

Use(s) and preparation: Malaria.

3-4 cups of an infusion made from 10 g of the leaves and 10 g of the leaves of *Lycopersicon* esculentum L. are drunk as a remedy for malaria.

Cymbopogon citratus (Nees) Stapf. (G070) (Image on page 191)

Vernacular: Obonyansi bw'echae

Use(s) and preparation: Fevers and colds.

3-4 cups of a decoction made from 10 g of the leaves are drunk daily

Eleusine coracana (L.) Gaertn (G071) (Image on page 194)

Vernacular name: Obori

Use(s) and preparation: Itchy rashes.

The flour is made into a paste and rubbed all over the body of a person suffering from itchy rashes.

Hordeum vulgare L. (G072) (Image on page 200)

Vernacular name: Engano

Use(s) and preparation: Malnutrition

The partially germinated grains are dried, ground into a powder, fermented, sweetened with honey, made into a porridge and drunk for nutrition.

Sorghum bicolor L.(G073) (Image on page 215)

Vernacular name: Amaemba.

Use(s) and preparation: Diarrhea.

Porridge made from its flour is recommended for anybody suffering from diarrhea.

Zea mays L. (G074) (Image on page 220)

Vernacular name: Ebando/Egetuma

Use(s) and preparation: Sores in the mouth and swellings of the feet

2-3 cups of a decoction made from 10 g of ash from burnt maize are drunk twice a day to treat sores in the mouth of a young child. 100 g of corn silk in 1 litre of water is drunk daily to reduce swellings of feet, especially in pregnant women.

LABIATAE

Ajuga remota Benth. (G075) (Image on page 183)

Vernacular name: Omosinyonta

Use(s) and preparation: Constipation

2-3 cups of a decoction made from 10 g of the leaves and 10 g of the stem are drunk. This is a useful treatment for constipation, especially in small children.

Leonotis nepetifolia R.Br.. (G076) (Image on page 202)

Vernacular name: Risibi rienyoni

Use(s) and preparation: Stomachache.

2-3 cups of an infusion made from 10 g of the leaves per litre of water are drunk.

Mentha piperita L. (G077) (Image on page 203)

Vernacular name: Mitisosi

Use(s) and preparation: Dyspepsia, intestinal gas, headaches and migraines, digestive colics, spasms, gastric atony, hepatitis and physical exhaustion, rheumatic and muscular aches.

3-4 cups of an infusion made from 20-40 g of the leaves in 1 litre are drunk daily.

Ocinum basilicum L. (G078) (Image on page 205)

Vernacular name: Ribuko

Use(s) and preparation: Insect repellant, stomach pains, constipation, nasal and bronchial catarrh.

2-3 cups of a decoction made from 30-40 g per litre of water are taken daily for stomach pains and constipation. 100 g of the leaves are boiled in water and the steam is inhaled for nasal and bronchial catarrh.

Ocimum kilimandscharicum Guerke (G079) (Image on page 204)

Vernacular name: Omote oitimo

Use(s) and preparation): Stomach problems, colds, coughs and measles.

2-3 cups of a decoction made from 50 g of leaves per litre of water are drunk three times daily as a remedy for stomach problems. 5-10 g of leaves are rubbed between the palms and sniffed as a remedy for colds and coughs. An infusion of 100 g of pounded leaves per litre of water is used as a water bath for the treatment of measles.

Ocimum lamiifolium Hochst ex Benth. (G080) (Image on page 205)

Vernacular name: Esurancha

Use(s) and preparation: Blocked nostrils, abdominal and stomach problems, sore eyes, earache and coughs.

5-10 g of fresh leaves are rubbed between the palms and sniffed as a remedy for blocked nostrils. 3-4 cups of a decoction made from 30-40 g of leaves of this plant and 30-40 g of the leaves of *Leonotis nepetifolia* per litre of water are drunk as a treatment for abdominal pains and stomach problems. An infusion made from 100 g of leaves in 1 litre of water is used as an eye wash, eardrops and 2-3 cups of the same infusion are drunk 3 times daily as a remedy for coughs.

Ocimum suave Willd. (G081) (Image on page 204)

Vernacular name: Omonyinkwa

Use(s) and preparation: Abdominal and stomach problems, sore eyes, earache and coughs.

2-3 cups of a decoction made from 30-40 g of leaves of this plant and 30-40 g of the leaves of *Leonotis nepetifolia* per litre of Water are drunk as a treatment for abdominal pains and stomach problems. An infusion made from 100 g of leaves in

1 litre of water is used as an eye Wash, eardrops and 2-3 cups of the same infusion are drunk 3 times daily as a remedy for coughs.

Orthosiphon hildebrandtii Benth. (G082) (Image on page 205)

Vernacular name: Ekebungabaiseke

Use(s) and preparation: Stomach problems.

3-4 cups of an infusion made from 10 g of leaves, 10 g of the leaves of *Ocimum suave* and 20 g of the leaves of *Leonotis nepetifolia* and mixed with 1 cup of fresh milk are drunk daily.

Plectranthus barbatus L'He'rit. (G083) (Image on page 208)

Vernacular name: Omoroka

Use(s) and preparation: Stomachache and measles.

2-3 cups of an infusion made from 20-30g of fresh leaves in 1 litre of water are drunk three times as a remedy for stomachache. 3-4 cups of the same infusion are drunk three times daily as a remedy for measles.

Rosmarinus officinalis L. (G084) (Image on page 211)

Vernacular name: Erosimeri.

Use(s) and preparation: stimulant, carminative, diaphoretic and flavouring agent.

2-3 cups of a decoction of 20-30 g of the dry and ground leaves made in 1 litre of water are drunk. 1 teaspoonful of the dry and ground leaves is mixed with the respective food recipes.

LAURACEAE

Persea gratissima (L.) Gaertn. (Syn *Persea americana* Miller) (exotic) (G085) (Image on page 207)

Vernacular name: Avocado

Use(s) and preparation: High blood pressure, pains, fever, diarrhea; headache, rheumatism and dysentery.

9-110 mashed seeds are boiled until they become a light paste. Arid 2-3 cups are drunk daily for headache, rheumatism, diarrhea and dysentery. 2-4 cups of a decoction made from 100 g of leaves in 1 litre of water are drunk three times daily for high blood pressure. An infusion made from 100 g of the leaves per litre of water is used in water baths for pain and fever.

LILIACEAE

Allium cepa L. (exotic) (G086) (Image on page 183)

Vernacular name: Egetunguo

Use(s) and preparation: Wound healing, furuncles, abscesses, helminths, rheumatism, arthritis and gouts.

5 g of onion is eaten raw, usually sliced or grated as a salad for the expulsion of intestinal worms. 1 bulb of onion is ground, and mixed with some honey and 1 cup is taken daily for rheumatism, arthritis and gouts. For good digestion, broth from cooked onions in any vegetable recipe is recommended. 2-3 cups are drunk daily after meals. For skin infections compresses soaked in onion juice are recommended. For the treatment of abscesses and furuncles hot boiled onion is applied directly on the affected area.

Allium sativum L. (exotic) (G087) (Image on page 183)

Vernacular name: Egetunguo saumu

Use(s) and preparation: Hypertension and earache.

Lemon juice is added to a macerate of 10 g of garlic, boiled and strained. The extract is drunk for hypertension. For an aching ear, a piece of garlic is boiled in coconut oil and used as eardrops.

Asparagus africanus Lam. (G088) (Image on page 184)

Vernacular name: Ekerobo

Use(s) and preparation: Boils.

5 g of the leaves are macerated and pasted on a boil to quicken their healing.

Gloriosa superba L. (G089) (Image on page 198)

Vernacular name: Omorero bwenyang'au

Use(s) and preparation: Abortion, indigestion, aphrodisiac and gouts.

2-3 cups of a decoction made from 10-15 g of root tissue per litre of water are drunk for abortion and for indigestion. 1 cup of an infusion made from 10-15 g of root tissue is drunk as an aphrodisiac and to treat gouts.

Warning: Little quantities should be taken at a time, as the plant rhizomes are poisonous.

MALVACEAE

Abutilon mauritiunum (Jacq.) Medic. (G090) (Image on page 181)

Vernacular name: Omorobianda

Usc(s) and preparation: Diarrhea, stomach cramps and bronchitis

2 cups of an infusion of 20-30 g of a dry powder of the leaves in 1 litre of Water are drunk daily for diarrhea. 2 cups of a decoction made from 20-30 of the root powder are drunk daily for stomach cramps and bronchitis.

Gossypium barbadense L. (exotic) (G091) (Image on page 198)

Vernacular name: Ebamba

Use(s) and preparation: Coughs, stomachache and constipation, earache and sores.

2 -3 cups of an infusion made from 10 g of fresh leaves per litre of Water are drunk for coughs. A decoction made from 20-30 g of leaves per litre of water is given to children for constipation. The juice from a warmed bud is squeezed into the ear for earache. The wool is used as padding and bandages for sores.

Gossypium herbaceum L. (exotic) (G092) (Image on page 199)

Vernacular name: Ebamba

Use(s) and preparation: Bronchial catarrh.

4 cups of an infusion made of 20 g of leaves, 20 g of flowers and a handful of seeds per litre of water are drunk daily.

Hibiscus fuscus Garcke (G093) (Image on page 199)

Vernacular name: Egesiringi

Use(s) and preparation: Tuberculosis, flu and whooping cough.

4-5 cups of a decoction of 30-40 g of 100 g of leaves in 1 litre of water are drunk for tuberculosis. 2-3 cups of a decoction of 100 g of flowers in 1 litre of water are drunk for flu and whooping cough.

Hibiscus rosa-sinensis L. (exotic) (G094) (Image on page 200

Vernacular name: Egesiringi ekiegarori

Use(s) and preparation: Intestinal pains, pile or kidney colic and dysmenorrhea.

2-3 cups of an infusion with 40-60g of seeds per litre of water are drunk daily

Sida cordifolia L. (G095) (Image on page 212)

Vernacular name: Ekerundu

Use(s) and preparation: Stimulates menstruation, and abortion

The bark is chewed to stimulate menstruation. As an abortifacient, the extract is drunk 3 times daily for two days.

Sida tenuicarpa Vollesen. (Syn *Sida cuinefolia* Cuf. non Roxb. (G096) (Image on page 212)

Vernacular name: Ekeburanchogu

Use(s) and preparation: Poison antidote, sore throat, quietening a fetus and wound healing.

100 g of dry leaves are ground into a powder 1 teaspoonful is pasted on an operated organ or part to remove poison. 1 cup of an infusion made from the powder drunk for sore throat. 1000 g of root material is boiled in 1 litre of water, strained, sweetened with honey and 1 cup is drunk three times to quieten a fetus which moves too much in the womb. A suitable quantity of the leaves/roots is macerated and pasted on a wound.

MELIACEAE

Ekebergia capensis Sparm. (G097) (Image on page 194)

Vernacular name: Omonyamari

Use(s) and preparation: Antihehminthic; dysentery.

3-4 cups of a decoction made from 10 g of bark material in 1 litre of water are drunk for dysentery and roundworms.

MELIANTHACEAE

Bersema abyssinica Fres. (G098) (Image on page 185)

Vernacular name: Omobamba

Use(s) and preparation: Expulsion of the placenta, colds; an aphrodisiac; Antihelmintic; dysentery and epilepsy.

3-4 cups of a decoction made from 10 g of root material are drunk to facilitate the expulsion of the placenta. Dry leaves are ground and used as a snuff for colds or chewed to act as an aphrodisiac. 2-3 cups of a decoction of 10 g of the powder of the dry bark are drunk against helminths. 3 cups of a decoction made from 10 g of young twigs are drunk for dysentery. 3 cups of a decoction made from 20 g of root material in 1 litre of water are drunk three times daily for epilepsy.

MIMOSACEAE

Acacia abyssinica Benth. ssp. *calophylla* Brenan (G099) (Image on page 181)

Vernacular name: Omonyenya omwegarori

Use(s) and preparation: Digestive problems and sore throat.

5 g of the gum is stirred in ½ a litre of honey and 1 cup of this mixture is drunk for digestive problems and sore throat.

Acacia nilotia (L.) Del. (G100) (Image on page 181)

Vernacular name: Omonyenya

Use(s) and preparation: Digestive problems and sore throat.

5 g of the gum is stirred in ½ a litre of honey and 1 cup of this mixture is drunk for digestive problems and sore throat.

Acacia sieberiana DC. (G101) (Image on page 182)

Vernacular name: Eyesura

Use(s) and preparation: Digestive problems and: sore throat.

5 g of the gum is stirred in ½ litre of honey and one cup of this mixture is drunk for digestive problems and sore throat.

Albizia gummifera (JF Gmel.) C.A. Sm.var. *gummifera* (G102) (Image on page 183)

Vernacular name: Omogonchoro

Use(s) and preparation: Digestive problems and sore throat.

5 g of the gum is stirred in ½ a litre of honey and one cup of this mixture is drunk during bedtime as a treatment for digestive problems and sore throat.

Mimosa pudica (L.) Del. (G103) (Image on page 203)

Vernacular name: Ekiebundi

Use(s) and preparation: Dysentery, diarrhea and sexually transmitted diseases.

2-3 cups of a decoction of 30-40 g of the whole plant in 1 litre are drunk for the treatment of dysentery. 3-4 cups of a strong decoction of 100 g of the Whole plant per litre of water are drunk for days for sexually transmitted diseases.

2-3 cups of a strong decoction of 100 g of the leaves, bud or bark in 1 litre of water are drunk for dysentery and diarrhea.

Ficus natalensis Hochst. (G104) (Image on page 196))

Vernacular name: Omogumo

Use(s) and preparation: Stomach problems and skin diseases

The leaves are burnt to ash. 2-3 spoonfuls of this ash are stirred in a cup of water and drunk three times for stomach problems. The same ash is mixed with animal fat and applied directly on an area afflicted with a skin disease.

Ficus sansibarica Warb. (G105) (Image on page 197)

Vernacular name: Omoko

Use(s) and preparation: Stomach problems and skin diseases.

2-3 spoonfuls of ash from burnt leaves are stirred in a cup of water and drunk three times for stomach problems. The same ash is mixed with animal fat and applied directly on an area afflicted with a skin disease. A decoction of the leaves made from 50 g of leaves in 5 litres of water is used to bathe the whole body as a treatment for skin afflictions.

Ficus sur Forssk (G106) (Image on page 197)

Vernacular name: Omoraa

Use(s) and preparation: Stomach problems.

2-3 spoonfuls of ash from burnt leaves are stirred in a cup of water and drunk three times daily.

Ficus exasperate Vahl. (G107) (Image on page 196)

Vernacular name: Omosenia/Risenia

Use(s) and preparation: Skin diseases.

Ash from burnt leaves is mixed with animal fat and applied directly on an area afflicted with a skin disease. A decoction of the leaves made from 50 g of leaves in 5 litres of water is used to bathe the whole body.

MUSACEAE

Musa paradisiaca subsp sapientum Kuntze (G108) (Image on page 204)

Vernacular name: Ritoke

Use(s) and preparation: Thrush.

1-2 spoonfuls of the ash 10 g of leaves combined with 5 porcupine spines are stirred in a ½ cup of water is (are) drunk for thrush.

MYRSINACEAE

Maesa lanceolate Forssk (G109) (Image on page 202)

Vernacular name: Omoterere

Use(s) and preparation: Diarrhea and dysentery.

1 cup of a decoction of 100 g of leaves in 1 litre of water is drunk every four hours until diarrhea or dysentery stops.

MYRTACEAE

Psidium guajava L. (exotic) (G110) (Image on page 209)

Vernacular name: Ripera

Use(s) and preparation: Diarrhea and dysentery.

1 cup of a decoction of 100 g of leaves in 1 litre of water is drunk every four hours until diarrhea or dysentery stops.

Eucalyptus globules Labill. (exotic) (G111) (Image on page 195)

Vernacular name: Omoringamu bw'amache

Use(s) and preparation: Insect repellants; bronchial catarrh, asthma, acute chronic bronchitis, colitis, diarrhea, intestinal problems, bad breath and fermentations.

50 g of fresh leaves are macerated and dropped into boiling water, steeped for 15 minutes sweetened with honey and 3 cups drunk after every meal for bronchial catarrh, asthma and acute and chronic bronchitis. 10 g of a handful of finely ground charcoal are(is) dissolved in water and 2-3 cups in cases of an emergency e.g. poisoning. 10 g of charcoal is stirred in 1 cup of water until a paste is formed. This is drunk two times daily for indigestion, diarrhea or intestinal fermentations. 1 teaspoonful of finely ground charcoal is taken one hour earlier before meals for bad breath.

Warning: Never exceed the recommended doses as this might lead to gastroenteritis and blood in the urine.

Eucalyptus camaldulensis Dennhardt. (Syn *Eucalyptus rostara* Schlechtendal (G112) (Image on page 195)

Vernacular name: Omoringamu omokong'u (kamu ngumu)

Use(s) and preparation: Bronchial catarrh, asthma, acute and chronic bronchitis, colitis, diarrhea, intestinal problems or fermentations.

50 g of fresh leaves are macerated and the macerate is dropped into boiling water and steeped for fifteen minutes, strained, and sweetened with honey. 3 cups of this extract are drunk daily after every meal as a remedy for bronchial catarrh, asthma and acute and chronic bronchitis.

OXALIDACEAE

Oxalis corniculata L. (G113) (Image on page 206)

Vernacular name: Enyonyo enene

Use(s) and preparation: Stomachache, inflamed eyelids, coughs, diarrhea and ringworms.

2 cups of an infusion made from 10g of leaves in 1 litre of water are drunk for stomachache. The same infusion is used as eye drops to cure an inflamed eyelid, cough and diarrhea.

A macerate of 10 g of the leaves is applied directly on an area infected with ringworms.

Oxalis latifolia L. (G114) (Image on page 206)

Vernacular name: Enyonyo

Use(s) and preparation: Inflamed rectum.

9 g of the leaves of this plant are combined with 10 g of the leaves of *Orthispon prophetarum* are macerated in 1 litre of water and strained and introduced into an inflamed rectum.

PALMAE

Phoenix reclinata Jacq. (G115) (Image on page 207)

Vernacular name: Rikendo

Use(s) and preparation: Skin diseases.

1 handful of fresh fruits is eaten daily.

Serenoa repens (Bartram) Small. (G116) (Image on page 212)

Vernacular name: Rikendo eriegarori

Use(s) and preparation: Cystitis, enlargement of the prostate glands and senile impotence

3-4 cups of a decoction made from 100 g of the powder of the ripe fruit in 1 litre of water are drunk daily.

PAPILIONACEAE

Arachis hypogea L. (exotic) (G117) (Image on page 184)

Vernacular name: Chinchugu

Use(s) and preparation: Dislocated joints

The oil is pressed from the seeds and then mixed with local gin and used as an ointment to massage dislocated joints or any organ where blood is not flowing freely.

Cajuns cajan (L.) Millsp. (G118) (Image on page 187)

Vernacular name: Chimbisi

Use(s) and preparation: Wounds, skin infections, ulcers, infected gums and toothache.

A decoction of 10 g of the leaves made in 1 litre of water is applied on wounds, skin infections and ulcers.

Crotalaria retusa L. (G119) (Image on page 190)

Use(s)and preparation: Wounds, skin infections and ulcers.

A decoction of 10 g of the leaves and 10 g of bark material made in 1 litre of water is applied on wounds, skin infections and ulcers.

Erythrina abyssinica DC. (G120) (Image on page 195)

Vernacular name: Omotembe

Use(s) and preparation: Trachoma, Antihelmintic, gonorrhea, syphilis, snake bite, and anthrax.

3 cups of the decoction made from 20 g finely ground bark and 10 g of the root tissue in 1 litre of water are drunk for the treatment of trachoma. The same decoction acts as a vermifuge. 3-4 cups of the same decoction are drunk for gonorrhea, syphilis and snake bite.

Indigofera arrecta A. Rich. (G121) (Image on page 200)

Vernacular name: Omocheo

Use(s) and preparation: Stomachache.

3-4 cups of an infusion made from 10 g of the roots in 1 litre of water are drunk.

Kotschya africana Endl. (G122) (Image on page 201)

Vernacular name: Omosing'oro

Use(s) and preparation: Stomach problems

3-4 cups of a decoction made from 10 g of the roots in 1 litre of water and drunk.

Phaseolus vulgaris L. (G123) (Image on page 207)

Vernacular name: Ching'ende

Use(s) and preparation: Edema, gout, kidney stones and premenstrual retention of fluid.

Green pods are cooked, dressed with oil and lemon juice and eaten as vegetables for edema, gout, kidney stones and premenstrual retention of fluid. A decoction with 100 g of dry bean pods in 1 litre of water is boiled until the liquid reduces to half its original volume and drunk daily edema and premenstrual retention of liquid.

Sesbania sesban (L.) Merrill var. *nubica* Chiov. (G124) (Image on page 212)

Vernacular name: Omosabisabi

Use(s) and preparation: Stomachache.

3-4 cups of an infusion made from 10 g of leaves in 1 litre of water are drunk as a remedy for stomachache.

Tephrosia nana Kotschy & Schweinf. (G125) (Image on page 216)

Vernacular name: Omochegechege

Use(s) and preparation: Indigestion, rheumatic fever, malaria fever and excessive thirst.

2-3 cups of a decoction made from 10 g of the root bark and 1 g of the powder of unripe pepper are drunk for indigestion, rheumatic fever, malaria fever and excessive thirst.

Vigna subterranean L. (G126) (Image on page 219)

Vernacular name: Chinchugu

Use(s) and preparation; Roots are chewed for the removal of the placenta in women.

2-3 cups of an infusion made from 20 g of roots in 1 litre of water are drunk for the removal of after-birth.

PASSIFLORACEAE

Passiflora incamata L. (Syn *Passiflora subpeltata* L.) (G127) (Image on page 207)

Vernacular name: Ritindogoro (Ritunda nyakoranda)

Use(s) and preparation: Anxiety, nervousness, insomnia, alcoholism and drug addiction.

An infusion of 20 g of the flowers and 20 g of the leaves is prepared in 1 litre of water, sweetened and drunk for insomnia. 50 g of flowers and 50 g of leaves are dropped into 1 litre of boiling water. The infusion is then decanted, sweetened with honey and 3 cups are drunk daily for alcoholism and drug withdrawal.

PIPERACEAE

Piper capense L. (G128) (Image on page 208)

Vernacular name: Ekenyanengo

Use(s) and preparation: Sore throat.

2 cups of a decoction made from 40 g of the roots in 1 litre of water are drunk daily for sore throat.

POLYGONACEAE

Oxygonum sinuatum (Hochst & Steud ex. Meisn) (G129) (Image on page 206)

Vernacular name: Omonyantira omwegarori

Use(s) and preparation: Boils, tonsillitis and sore eyes

A handful of leaves are macerated and the macerate is pasted on a boil to make it ripen faster so that the pus can be squeezed out to hasten healing. A decoction made from 30 g in 1 litre of water is gargled as a remedy for tonsillitis. 10 g of the leaves are macerated and the extract is used as eye drops to treat a diseased eye.

Rumex usambarensis (Dammer) Dammer. (G130) (Image on page 211)

Vernacular name: Omonyantira

Use(s) and preparation: Malaria, TB, wound healing and scabies.

20 g of the whole plant is burnt into ashes. 2-3 spoonfuls of this ash are stirred in a cup of honey and drunk as a treatment for malaria and tuberculosis (TB). 10 g of the whole plant is combined with 10 g of the leaves of *Ajuga remota* and then burnt to ashes. Two to three spoonfuls of this ash are stirred in a cup of honey and applied directly to wounds to quicken their healing. A decoction made from 50 g of the leaves in 1 litre of water is used as a bath for the body of a person suffering from scabies.

PROTEACEAE
Fauera rochetiana (A. Rich.) Pic. Ser. (G131) (Image on page 196)
Vernacular name: Omosasa

Use(s) and preparation: Expulsion of intestinal parasites.

15 g of the powder of the rhizome and the root are swallowed. For children, the dose should be halved.

Warning: During the treatment, no alcoholic beverages should be taken. No more than 10 g of the powder should be swallowed.

Faurea saligna Harr. (G132) (Image on page 196)
Vernacular name: Omosasa omwegaroi

Use(s) and preparation: Malaria and venereal diseases.

3-4 cups of a decoction made from 15-20 g of the roots in 1 litre of water are drunk daily.

RHAMNACEAE
Rhamnus staddo A. Rich. (G133) (Image on page 210)
Vernacular name: Omonyanengo

Use(s) and preparation: Malaria and venereal diseases.

3-4 cups of a decoction made from 20-30 g of the leaves and 15-20 g of the roots in 1 litre of water are drunk daily.

Rhamnus prinoides L' He'rit. (G134) (Image on page 209)

Vernacular name: Omong'ura

Use(s) and preparation: Indigestion, gonorrhea, malaria and rheumatism

3-4 cups of a decoction made from 100 g of ground roots in 1 litre of water are drunk daily.

ROSACEAE

Fragaria vesca L. (G135) (Image on page 198)

Vernacular name: Chinkenene

Use(s) and preparation: Arthritis and gouts.

2-3 kg of ripe fruit is eaten daily with no other food except water.

Hagennia abyssinica (Bruce) J.F.) Gmel. (G136) (Image on page 199)

Vernacular name: Omokunakuna

Pirus malus L. (exotic) (G137) (Image on page 208)

Vernacular name: Riembe

Use(s) and preparation: Diarrhea, colitis, dysentery, constipation, arthritis, rheumatism, gout, kidney stones, digestive and respiratory afflictions, and high blood pressure. For any diarrhea, ½ kg of grated raw apples and also roasted or boiled should be eaten daily. After thorough cleaning. For arthritis, rheumatism, gout and kidney stones, a decoction of two sliced apples in 1 litre of water sweetened with honey is recommended. 1 cup is drunk three times daily, for kidney stones or sand, kidney inflammation and arterial hypertension, a decoction of 50 g of leaves and 50 g flowers made in 1 litre of water is recommended. 3-4 four cups are drunk daily to act as a diuretic.

Prunus africana (Hook. f.) Kalkm. (Syn *Pygeum africana* Hook. f.) (G138) (Image on page 209)

Vernacular name: Ekeburabura

Use(s) and preparation: Purgative and prostate gland problems.

2 cups of an infusion of 10-20 g of the dried and ground bark made in 1 litre of water are drunk.

RUBIACEAE

Coffea Arabica L. (exotic) (G139) (Image on page 189)

Vernacular name: Ekagwa

Use(s) and preparation: Central nervous stimulant, an aphrodisiac, alcoholic intoxication, blackouts and fainting due to physical exhaustion and tiredness, headaches, migraines, fever and head congestion clue to influenza.

2-3 cups of an infusion of green or toasted fruits that are finely ground are drunk daily.

Rubia cordifolia L. (G140) (Image on page 211)

Vernacular name: Eng'urang'uria

Use(s) and preparation: stomachache, antidote for general poisoning, diarrhea and skin rashes.

3 cups of a decoction made from 10 g of the roots in 1 litre of water are drunk for the treatment of stomachache. These are drunk 3 times daily. 2 cups of a decoction made from 10 g of the leaves and 10 g of the stem in 1 litre of water are drunk for the treatment of diarrhea. Two cups of a decoction made from 10 g of the leaves in 1 litre of water are drunk daily for the treatment of skin rashes.

Rytigynia acuminatissima (K. Schum) Robyns (G141) (Image on page 212)

Vernacular name: Omonyiinga

Use(s) and preparation: Stomachache, intestinal worms, and scurvy.

2-3 cups of an infusion made from 10 g of macerated leaves in 1 litre of water are drunk as a remedy for stomachache. 5 cups of a decoction made from 15 g of roots in 1 litre of water are drunk as a remedy for intestinal worms. The fruits are also eaten as a preventative measure against scurvy.

Vangueria apiculata K. Schum. (G142) (Image on page 218)

Vernacular name: Omokomoni

Use(s)and preparation: Stomachache, intestinal worms and, and scurvy.

3 cups of an infusion made from 10 g of macerated leaves are drunk as a remedy for stomachache. 5 cups of a decoction made from 15 g of roots in 1 litre of water are drunk as a remedy for intestinal worms. The fruits are also eaten as a preventative measure against scurvy.

RUTACEAE

Citrus aurantium L. (*Citrus limon* (L.) Burn. (exotic) (G143) (Image on page 189)

Vernacular name: Ritunda riroro

Use(s) and preparation: Insomnia, migraine, stomach spasms and nerves in the stomach, belching, fishing, heart palpitations, fainting and weakness of fatigue, menstrual pain, edema, hemorrhages, a digestive tonic, appetizer, indigestion and a sedative.

30 g of the leaves and 30 g of the flowers are made into an infusion in 1 litre of water. 3-4 cups are drunk daily when retiring to bed. This brings on sleep quickly, 50 g of dry rind is cut into pieces and then boiled for 30 minutes, sweetened with honey and a cup of this decoction is drunk daily after each meal as a remedy for edema, indigestion and varicose veins.

Clausena anisata (Willd.) Benth. (G144) (Image on page 189)

Vernacular name: Omonyansuri

Use(s) and preparation: Coughs and stomachaches and paralysis

1 cup of the decoction made from 15 g of roots in 1 litre of water is drunk for the treatment of coughs and stomachaches. A root infusion made from 1 litre of water is put into incisions and some of this decoction is taken orally as a remedy for paralysis caused by snakebite.

Toddalia asiastica (L.) Lam. (G145) (Image on page 217)

Vernacular name: Ekenagwa ekiagarori

Use(s) and preparation: Coughs, colds and stomachaches.

2-3 cups of a decoction made from 15 g of the roots in 1 litre of water are drunk for the coughs and stomachaches.

SOLANACEAE

Capsicum frutescens L. (G146) (Image on page 187)

Vernacular name: Earare

Use(s) and preparation: Palpitations, asthma, cough and cold in the chest, boils, nausea, indigestion or, sore throat, bloated stomach, lack of appetite, rheumatism, lumbago, stiff neck and muscular aches.

The fruit is cooked as a vegetable in any cooking recipe to act as a remedy for those suffering from a bloated stomach or slow digestion and from lack of appetite. Small doses are recommended. It can also be sprinkled on food in the form of a dry powder. Poultices of hot peppers are applied on aching parts or areas. These apes are then covered with a woollen cloth.

Warning: People suffering from severe stomachaches must abstain from eating hot peppers.

Datura arborea L (G147) (Image on page 192)

Vernacular name: Ekeroria

Use(s) and preparation: Stomachache and gall bladder pain.

Leaves are ground in and soaked in water for a day in tablespoonfuls (100 ml) of water and are drunk 3 times daily. (10-15 drops after 4 hours for adults only.

Warning: *Datum arborea* is very poisonous if more than the recommended dosage is taken.

Datura stramonium L. (G148) (Image on page 192)

Vernacular name: Ekeroro

Use(s) and preparation: Asthma, colic pains and rheumatism.

Dry leaves are ground into a fine powder, and a small quantity of this is rolled into a cigarette and smoked for the treatment of asthma and colic pains. Dry leaves are macerated and mixed with maize flour until a paste is formed. This paste is made into a poultice and applied to affected parts to ease rheumatic pains.

Warning: This is a very toxic plant. It must not at all be used internally.

Nicotiana tabacum L. (exotic) (G149) (Image on page 204)

Vernacular name: Etumbato

Use(s) and preparation: Colds, emetic, and nervous tension.

Fingertip of the dried and ground leaves is placed in the nostrils of a person with a cold. This is to promote sneezing (sternutatory). The dry leaves are ground and placed on fresh wounds to stop bleeding. The ground leaves are also mixed with animal ghee and applied on an area infected with ringworm.

Solanum acueastrum Dunal (G150) (Image on page 213)

Vernacular name: Omotobo

Use(s) and preparation: Diarrhea, gonorrhea, vomiting, toothache, syphilis and abdominal pains.

50 g of root material per 250 ml of water is made into a decoction. 1 cup of this decoction drunk three times daily as a treatment for gonorrhea, vomiting, toothache, syphilis and abdominal pains.

Solanum incanum L. (G151) (Image on page 213)

Vernacular name: Omoratora

Use(s) and preparation: Tonsillitis, muscular cramps, diarrhea, gonorrhea, vomiting, toothache, syphilis, abdominal, pains, and snakebite.

20 g of the burnt ash is mixed with animal fat and with the help of a piece of a clean cloth, this mixture is rubbed on an area affected with swellings brought about as a result of tonsillitis. 1 cup of a decoction made from 50 g of roots and 50 g of leaves in 1 litre of water is drunk three times daily after every meal as a remedy for muscular cramps. 50 g of root material per 250 ml of water is made into an infusion. 1 cup of this infusion is drunk three times daily as a treatment for gonorrhea, vomiting, toothache, syphilis and abdominal pains.

Solanum mauense Bitter. (G152) (Image on page 214)

Vernacular name: Engeng'encha

Use(s) and preparation: The root decoction is used as a remedy for malaria and chest pains.

2-3 cups of a root decoction made from 100 g in 1 litre of water are drunk daily.

Solanum mauritianum Scop. (G153) (Image on page 214)

Vernacular name: Omonsarigo

Use(s) and preparation: Itching in the vagina, or arms, scabies, ringworm and herpes.

Lotions with the fresh juice of the leaves and stems are applied directly to the affected parts.

Solanum nigrum L. (G154) (Image on page 214)

Vernacular name: Rinagu

Use(s) and preparation: Itching in the vagina or the arms, scabies, ringworm

Lotions with the fresh juice of the leaves and stems are applied directly to the affected parts. Poultices with the mashed leaves are applied directly on the affected parts.

TILIACEAE

Triumfetta branchyceras K. Schum. (Syn *Triumfetta macrophylla* K. Schum.) (G155) (Image on page 218)

Vernacular name: Ekemiso

Use(s) and preparation: Constipation, indigestion problems, minor pains and aching in newborns.

50-60 g of the powder of the dry leaves are mixed with 1 litre of water. 3-4 cups are drunk daily for constipation and other indigestion problems. 100 g of fresh leaves are pounded and mixed with 2 litres of water. This infusion is used to bathe newborn babies. This acts as a remedy for itching. For minor pains, the same water can be used as a bath.

Triumfetta rhomboidea Jacq. (G156) (Image on page 218)

Vernacular name: Omomiso

Use(s) and preparation: Facilitation of first purching in newborns, burns, toothache and circumcision wounds.

1 cup of a decoction made from 5 g of the closed flowers in 1 litre of water is given to newborn babies to facilitate the first patching. The leaves are macerated and the macerate is then pasted on wounds resulting from burns to quicken their healing. A root infusion made from 30 g of root material in 1 litre of water is used as a gargle to treat toothache. The same infusion is applied to circumcision wounds to hasten their healing,

Corchorus olitorius L. (G157) (Image on page 190)

Vernacular name: Omotere

Use(s) and preparation: Increases milk production in women

Cooked with any vegetable recipe and eaten.

THEACEAE

Thea sinensis L. (G158) (Image on page 216)

Vernacular name: Echae

Use(s) and preparation: Stimulant, diarrhea, colitis, a digestive tonic, and conjunctivitis

30-50 g of dried and ground tea are dropped into 1 litre of boiling water. 4-5 cups of this infusion are drunk daily as a cure for diarrhea, colitis, upset stomach or indigestion. 40-60 g of dried and ground leaves are dropped into 1 litre of water. This is boiled for 10 minutes allowed to cool, and then applied to the eye as eye drops to treat conjunctivitis.

ULMACEAE

Trema orientalis (L). Bl. (G159) (Image on page 217)

Vernacular name: Omonyia

Use(s) and preparation: Demulcent and emollient

100-200 g of the powdered drug is mixed with 1 litre of water. This is boiled and mixed with cassava flour and stirred to make a paste. This paste is used as a poultice and applied on dislocated joints.

UMBELLIFERAE

Daucus carota L. (G160) (Image on page 192)

Vernacular name: Ekarati

Use(s) and preparation: Conjunctivitis, ulcers, diarrhea and colitis, wounds, burns, eczema, acne, abscesses, Induction of menstruation and avoidance of intestinal gases.

Raw carrots, sliced or shredded, are eaten to improve vision. The juice can also be drunk immediately after preparation, alone or mixed with lemon and/or apple juice. This is still for the improvement of vision. The juice must be drunk over long periods to produce its beneficial effects. Herbal tea with carrot seeds (40-50 g per litre of water) is recommended for the treatment of stomachaches and any excess acidity. For the treatment of infected wounds, burns, eczema, acne, and abscesses poultices of cooked and mashed carrots are directly applied to the affected area.

Petroselimum crispum (Mill) Nyman. (Syn *Petroselinum sativum* Hoffman) (G161) (Image on page 207)

Vernacular name: Endania

Use(s) and preparation: Amenorrhoea, dysmenorrhoea, diuresis and a condiment for flavouring food.

2-3 cups of ripe fruit in 1 litre of water are drunk daily as a remedy for amenorrhoea and dysmenorrhoea and to induce diuresis. It is also used as a condiment.

URTICACEAE

Urtica dioica L. (G162) (Image on page 218)

Vernacular name: Rise

Use(s) and preparation: Rheumatic afflictions, gout, arthritis, kidney stones, urinary sand, malnutrition, fatigue, for women with excessive malnutrition, uterine and nasal hemorrhages, digestive disorders, diarrhea, colitis, dysentery, eczema, eruptions, acne and loss of hair.

30-40 g of fresh whole plant material is macerated in 1 litre of water and then strained using sackcloth. 1 cup of the resulting extract is drunk two times daily as a treatment for rheumatism, gout, arthritis, kidney stones and urinary sand. An infusion made from 50 g of fresh whole plant material per litre of water is steeped for 1 hour and 4 cups of this are drunk daily, preferably after every meal as a remedy for gout, rheumatism, arthritis, kidney stones, and urinary sand, uterine and nasal haemorrhages. Juice from the whole plant is applied on an area afflicted with eczema, eruptions, acne or hair loss. Compresses, soaked in juice made from an infusion of whole plant material, usually 100 g in 1 litre of water, are applied to an area affected by eczema, eruptions and acne. These compresses are changed five times daily. In the case of nasal haemorrhages cotton wool is soaked in the above juice and plugged into the nostrils. For the treatment of a rheumatic or inflammatory disorder, a freshly gathered bunch of the plant is used to gently hit the skin of the affected joint e.g. knee, shoulder, etc. This causes a revulsive effect to take place. This action attracts blood to the skin, thus decongesting the internal tissues.

VERBENACEAE

Lantana camara L. (G163) (Image on page 201)

Vernacular name: Obori bw 'enyoni

Use(s) and preparation: Abortifacient, stomachache, malaria, rheumatism, coughs, sore throat, toothache, conjunctivitis, colds, headache and itching.

3-4 cups of an infusion made from 20 g of leaves per litre of water are for migraines. A decoction of 30 g in 1 litre of water is allowed to stand for 1 hour and 1 cup is drunk after every meal as for coughs, sore throat colds and headaches. For sinusitis, the patient's steam from the hot decoction is inhaled. Hot compresses of a concentrated infusion or decoction are applied to the affected parts. Throat afflictions can also be healed by the use of poultices of a stewed plant wrapped in cotton fabric.

Lappia javanica (Burm.f.) Spreng. (G164) (Image on page 201)

Vernacular name: Omonyinkwa

Use(s) and preparation: Antiseptic

A decoction made of 50-60 g of root tissue in 1 litre of water is used as an antiseptic.

VITACEAE

Rhoicissus tridentate (G165) (Image on page 210)

Vernacular name: Omonyambeche/Egesanga

Use(s) and preparation: Antiseptic.

A decoction made of 50-60 g of stem tissue in 1 litre of water is used as an antiseptic.

ZINGIBERACEAE

Zingiber officinale Roscoe (G166) (Image on page 220)

Vernacular name: Entangausi

Use(s) and preparation: Exhaustion, lack of appetite, bloated stomach, and flatulence.

Used for seasoning in small amounts for raw and uncooked food. 1 cup of an infusion of 2 g in 500 ml of water is drunk after every meal for all the above conditions.

Chapter Four

Antimicrobial Screening

4.1 Material and Methods

The plants used in this investigation were selected from the results of the ethnomedical survey. The criteria used for their selection were based on the revelation from the survey that they were widely used in the community for the treatment of infectious diseases of bacterial and fungal origin such as diarrhea, dysentery, ringworm, etc., Table 2 was generated from the responses of 1100 practicing traditional medical practitioners i.e. both small scale and large scale and large scale healers from the eleven divisions comprising the two districts. (Figures 1 c and 1 d). After the survey and having identified the 166 plant species from each traditional practitioner, a list was then sent to the same practitioners containing all the plants that had been identified in the survey. The traditional medical

practitioners were asked to pick twenty plants from the list that they frequently used in their medical practice. From these responses, Table 2 Was generated. The extracts of these plants were tested against the standard antibiotics that are listed in Table 1.

The microorganisms used in this investigation are listed in Table 3. They are representative microorganisms from gram-positive and gram-negative species. They were stock cultures preserved in the Department of Botany, Kenyatta University. They were transferred to new slants every two weeks. They will be referred to as local cultures. Clinical isolates obtained from Kenyatta National Hospital, and listed in Table 4, were also used. These were organisms that had been isolated from patients who had complicated clinical cases. The cultures were lyophilized and stored at 4°C until the time of use. These will be referred to as clinical isolates and reference cultures.

TABLE 1

List of reference antibiotics tested against stock cultures and clinical isolates and reference cultures

Antibiotic	Abbreviation	Micrograms
Ampicillin	Amp	25
Tetracycline	Tet	25
Cotrimoxazole	Cot	25
Kanamycin	Kan	30
Chloramphenicol	Chl	30
Amikacin	Amik	20
Cephalosporin	Ceph	10
Gentamycin	Gen	10

TABLE 2

List of medicinal plants commonly used selected from the ethnomedical survey based on the responses of 1100 traditional medical practitioners (n=1100= 100%)

Family	Species	% Response
Amaranthaceae	*Achyranthes aspera* L.	2
Caesalpinaceae	*Cassia occidentalis* L.	5
Compositae	*Ageratum conyzoides* L.	3
Compositae	*Bidens grantii* (Oliv.) Sherff-	4
Compositae	*Bidens pilosa* L.	2
Compositae	*Vernonia auriculifera* (Welw) Hiern.	35
Compositae	*Crassocephalum vitellinum* (Benth.) S. Moore.	4
Compositae	*Tagetes minuta* L.	5
Compositae	*Dicrocephala integrifialia* (L.f.) Kuntze.	2
Euphorbiaceae	*Euphorbia hirta* L.	6
Malvaceae	*Hibiscus fuscus* Garcke.	12
Papilionaceae	*Indigofera arrecta* A. Rich.	5
Verbenaceae	*Lantana camara* L.	2
Labiatae	*Ocimum basilicum* L.	4
Myrtaceae	*Psidium guajava* L.	7

Anacardiaceae	*Rhus vulgaris* Meikle.	6
Malvaceae	*Sida tenuicarpa,* Vollesen.*Sida cuinefolia*	5
Solanaceae	*Solanum incanum,* L.	9
Tiliaceae	*Triumfetta brachyceras* K. Schum.	3

TABLE 3

List of bacteria and fungi used during the screening of plant extracts for the anti-microbial activity of the selected medicinal plants

Bacteria	Characteristics
Streptococcus faecalis	Gram-positive coccus exists in chains and is a normal inhabitant of human intestines.
Escherichia coli	Gram-negative rod, facultative anaerobe and produces red pigments on nutrient agar.
Pseudomonas aeruginosa	Gram-negative rod causes opportunistic infections in man and is widely distributed in nature.
Streptococcus aureus	Gram-positive coccus, aerobic and widely distributed in nature.
Bacillus subtilis	Gram-positive rod, aerobic and spore-forming. It is widely distributed in the soil.
Enterobacter aerogenes	Gram-negative rod, facultatively anaerobic and widely distributed in the soil.
Proteus vulgaris	Gram-negative rod, motile. It is a normal intestinal flora but is also widely distributed in soil and water.
Candida albicans	Is a fungus and is gram-negative. It is widely distributed in nature and causes several infections in man and other animals.

TABLE 4

List of clinical isolates and reference cultures obtained from Kenyatta National Hospital and their clinical significance according to Jawetz et al. (1970)

Organism	Characteristics
Pseudomonas aeruginosa ATCC 28783	Is only a pathogen when introduced in areas devoid of normal defences and when participating in mixed infections. It produces infections of wounds, meningitis and urinary tracts. The micro-organism is resistant to most antimicrobial agents (produces Portent β-lactase. It is common in patients with leukemia or lymphoma who have received anti-neoplastic drugs or radiation and in severe burns
Escherichia coli ATCC 25922	These are normally organisms of the intestinal flora. They become pathogenic when they reach the tissues outside the intestinal tract, particularly the urinary tract, peritoneum or meninges where they cause inflammation when the immune system is impaired, or in early infancy or old age, they may reach the bloodstream and cause sepsis.
Vibro cholera (ogagwa) K017	The organism is very pathogenic to man. It is localized in the intestinal tract but liberates endotoxins, mucinaces and cholegen, which cause severe diarrhea, dehydration, acidosis, shock and death.
Salmonella typhi K012	This organism causes oral route infections called enteric fevers. The organism when ingested with contaminated food reaches the small intestines, then the intestinal lymphatics, where it causes necrosis of lymphoid tissue, liver and inflammation of the gall bladder.
Salmonella typhimurium K012	Produces gastroenteritis often called food poisoning. It causes local violent irritation of the mucous membranes. There is usually no invasion of the bloodstream and no distribution to other organs.

Proteus *rettigeri* *Proteus* *mirabilis* K039	These are free-living micro-organisms mainly in water, soil and sewage. Some species e. g. P. *vulgaris* commonly occur in normal faecal flora of the intestinal tracts. P. *morganis* has been incriminated in diarrhea in children. The two species, *P. rettigeri* and *P. Mirabilis* were chosen to represent this group.
Shigella *flaxineri* *Shigella* *boydii* *Shigella* *sonnei* *Shigella* *dysentery* K008 K032 K018 K019	The natural habitat of the dysentery bacilli is the large intestines of man. *Shigella* species infections are practically limited to the gastrointestinal tract. Bloodstream invasion is quite rare. Pathogenesis includes inflammation of the wall of the large intestines leading to necrosis of the mucous membrane.
Citrobacter *dweisus* K006	These organisms resemble *Salmonella* species, both in biochemical features and occasionally in pathogenicity in man.
Streptoccus *pyogenes* ATCC581899	The organism is one of the beta haemolytic varieties and causes streptococcal sore throat. In infants and small children, it causes subacute nasopharyngitis. In older children and adults, the disease is more acute and is characterized by intense nasopharyngitis, tonsillitis and edema of the mucous membrane.

(a) Extraction of *Euphorbia hirta* L.

In this preliminary screening of Euphorbia hirta L. the plant was separated into its various major parts i.e. roots, stems, leaves and flowers. Each part was dried and then ground to a powder. The resulting powder was kept in dark properly stoppered and sealed glass containers with printed labels and stored in a dark, cool and dry cupboard in the research awaiting extraction.

Fifty grams of the selected plant material was first extracted with the lipophilic solvent i.e. diethyl ether. After this the vegetable product was extracted using methanol (an intermediate polar solvent) and finally with water (a strong polar solvent). Three extracts were thus obtained i.e. the ether extract (E), the methanol extract (M) and the extract (W).

(I) The ether extract.

50 g of each powdered plant part (roots, stems, leaves and flowers) material was placed in a sample thimble of the Soxhlet apparatus and the 500 ml extraction flask filled with 400 ml of redistilled diethyl ether. The extraction process took 10 hours or until the extract was clear. This was then concentrated on a rotary evaporator at 50°C and the resulting concentrated sample was transferred to clean sterile sample bottles. This was further dried under vacuum over anhydrous copper sulphate to give a dry solid or paste of the extract for the bioassay.

(ii) The methanol extract

Fifty grams of each powdered plant material was placed in the sample thimble of the Soxhlet apparatus and the 500 ml extraction flask filled with 400 ml of the redistilled methanol (the redistillation was done twice to obtain the purified form). The extraction procedure took 10 hours or until the extract was clear. This was then concentrated on a rotary evaporator at 50°C and the resulting concentrated sample was transferred to clean sterile sample bottles. This was further dried under vacuum over anhydrous copper sulphate to give a dry solid or paste of the extract for the bioassay.

(iii) The water extract

Fifty grams of the powdered plant material was placed in 250 ml. Erlenmeyer flask and soaked in distilled water to a depth of about 4 cm above the surface. The flasks were then plugged with cotton wool to stop environmental contamination. This was shaken in the dark for 24 hours on a Jankee and Kunkel shaker set at 188 strokes per minute. The resulting aqueous extract was then suction-filtered and the process repeated until all soluble compounds had been extracted, as judged by loss of colour of the filtrate. Filtration Was done through Whatman filter paper No. 1. The filtrate was freeze-dried and then used for the bioassay.

b) The Bioassay

The test bacteria were inoculated in nutrient broth and the cultures were incubated at 35⁰C for 24 hours. *Candida albicans*, the test fungus, was inoculated in Potato dextrose agar broth and incubated under the same conditions as the bacterial cultures. The disc diffusion method was used for the preliminary antimicrobial screening. A concentration of 10 mg/ml of each crude extract was used.

A 24-hour culture of the test organism was swabbed onto the surface of the prepared sensitest agar and allowed to soak for five minutes. Sterile, soaked and dried sample discs were applied onto the surface of the inoculated sensitest agar, pressed firmly and allowed to diffuse slowly into the agar. Six discs impregnated with ether, methanol and water extracts, respectively for the root, stems, leaves and flowers were placed on each plate. Each test was done in duplicate. Control discs impregnated with an equal volume of ether, methanol and water were dried and also placed on the inoculated sensitest agar. All inoculated plates were incubated at 35°C for 24 hours. The diameter of inhibition was measured 24 hours after the growth of the organism. An average of the readings was then taken. Each reading was an average of six replicates

(c)Testing of extracts from the twenty selected medicinal plants against stock cultures and clinical isolates (or reference cultures) from Kenyatta National Hospital

For the other 19 plant species, the methanol extracts used were prepared following the same method as the one used for **E. hirta**

4.2 Results

The results are presented in Tables 5, 6, 7, 8, 9 and 10.

(i) Zones of inhibition (in mm) of reference antibiotics

The results of the above tests are summarized in Table 5. The interpretation of the results was done by the use of a zone-size interpretation chart devised by Bauer *et al.* (1966) whereby the inhibition zones of each antibiotic are judged separately and not compared to one another. According to this method of interpretation, only rational concentrations of antibiotics should be employed which can be related to systemic therapeutic levels. According to this method, a zone of inhibition of more than 6 mm and less than 11 mm was designated or thought of as the exhibition of slight activity; 12-17 mm was designated as intermediate activity and a zone of inhibition of 18 mm or more was designated sensitive.

According to the above interpretation S. *faecalis*, E. *coli*, and P. *aeruginosa* were resistant to ampicillin. S. *aureus*, E. *aerogenes* and P. *vulgaris* showed slight activity. B. *subtilis* showed intermediate response whereas C. *albicans* was sensitive to ampicillin.

P. *aeruginosa* is resistant to tetracycline, P. *vulgaris*, and C. *albicans* show a slight response whereas E. *coli* shows an intermediate response. S. *faecalis*, S. *aureus* B. *subtilis* and E. *aerogenes* are sensitive to this antibiotic. B. *subtilis* is resistant to cotrimoxazole. This antibiotic shows slight activity against P. *aeruginosa* and P. *vulgaris* whereas S. E. *coli*, S. *aureus*, E. *aerogenes* and C. *albicans* are sensitive to this antibiotic.

Kanamycin shows slight activity against P. *aeruginosa*, intermediate activity against B. *subtilis* and is sensitive to S. *faecalis*, E. *coli*, S. *aureus*, P. *aerogenes*, P. *vulgaris* and C. *albicans*. P. *aeruginosa* is resistant to chloramphenicol. This antibiotic shows slight activity against E. *aerogenes* and P. *vulgaris*. S. *faecalis*, E. *coli*, S. *aureus*, B. *subtilis* and C. *albicans* are sensitive to this antibiotic.

All the stock cultures that were tested against amikacin showed a sensitive response. Cephalosporin showed slight activity against S. *faecalis*, E. *coli*, P. *aeruginosa* and E. *aerogenes*. P. *vulgaris* showed intermediate activity whereas S. *aureus*, B. *subtilis* and C. *albicans* showed sensitivity to this antibiotic.

Gentamycin showed slight activity against E. *aeragenes*, and intermediate activity against P. *vulgaris*, and P. *aeruginosa*. S. *faecalis*, E. *coli*, S, *aureus*, B. *subtilis* and C. *albicans* showed sensitivity to this antibiotic. For S. *faecalis*, of the eight antibiotics that it was tested against, it was resistant to ampicillin, showed slight response to cephalosporin whereas it was sensitive to all the other antibiotics that showed zones of inhibition of more than 18 mm. For *E. coli* of the eight antibiotics that it was tested against, it was resistant to ampicillin, showed a slight response to cephalosporin and an intermediate response to tetracycline and was sensitive to cotrimoxazole, kanamycin, chloramphenicol, amikacin and gentamycin.

P. *aerugizrosa* was resistant to ampicillin, tetracycline and chloramphenicol. It showed a slight response to cotrimoxazole, kanamycin and cephalosporin. An intermediate response was shown towards gentamycin Whereas sensitivity was shown to amikacin. *S. aureus* showed a slight response to ampicillin and was sensitive to tetracycline, cotrimoxazole, kanamycin, chloramphenicol, amikacin, cephalosporin and gentamycin. *S. subtilis* was resistant to cotrimoxazole but showed an intermediate response to ampicillin and kanamycin and was sensitive to tetracycline, chloramphenicol, amikacin, cephalosporin and gentamycin.

E. aerogenes showed a slight response to ampicillin, chloramphenicol, cephalosporin and gentamycin but it was sensitive to tetracycline, cotrimoxazole, kanamycin and amikacin. *P. vulgaris* showed a slight response to ampicillin, tetracycline, cotrimoxazole and chloramphenicol. An intermediate response was shown to cephalosporin and gentamycin and sensitivity was shown to kanamycin and amikacin. *C. albicans* showed a slight response to tetracycline but it was sensitive to the rest of the seven antibiotics that it was tested against.

Results in Table 5 showed that antibiotics used as positive controls exhibited good inhibition of the growth of the stock bacterial species used. The range of inhibition was from 6.1 mm. to 29.2 mm as shown in Table 5. The lowest zone of inhibition was shown by ampicillin in three bacterial species namely *S. faecalis, E. coli* and *P. aeruginosa* ($F_{7, 49} = 2.99$, $P < 0.001$).

The results in Table 5 also show that amikacin was the most inhibitory antibiotic with inhibition zones ranging from 18.1 mm. to 29.2 mm. From the results, it can be seen that the most sensitive micro-organism was S. aureus and the least sensitive micro-organism was P. *aeruginosa*. This finding was statistically significant at ($F_{1, 49} = 2.99$, $P < 0.001$). The most sensitive micro-organism, *S. aureus* had zones of inhibition of more than 22 mm in six of the antibiotics that it was tested against.

(ii) Zones of inhibition (in mm) of reference antibiotics tested against clinical isolates obtained from Kenyatta National Hospital

The results of the above tests are summarized in Table 6. According to the interpretation of the zone-size chart by the method devised by Bauer *et al.* (1966) *P. rettigeri, S. flaxineri* and *S. pyogenes* were resistant to ampicillin. This antibiotic showed slight activity against *E. coli, P. aeruginosa, V. cholera, S. typhi, S. typhimirium, S. boydii, S. sonnei, S. dysenterica, C. dweisus* and *P. mirabilis*.

Resistance to tetracycline was shown by S. typhi and S. boydii. This antibiotic exhibited slight activity against *P. aeruginosa, V. cholera, S. typhimirium, S. flaxineri, P. rettigeri, S. sonnei, S. dysenterica, C. dweisus and P. mirabilis, E. coli* and *S. pyogenes* were sensitive to this antibiotic. Four pathogens, namely *P. aeruginosa, V. cholera, S. flaxineri,* and *P. mirabilis* were resistant to cotrimoxazole. This antibiotic showed slight activity against *S. typhi, P. rettigeri* and *C. dweisus*. Intermediate activity was shown towards *S. sonnei, E. coli, S. boydii, S. dysenterica* and *S. pyagenes* were sensitive to this antibiotic.

P. aeruginosa showed resistance to kanamycin. This antibiotic showed slight activity against *V. cholera, S. typhi, S. typhimurium, P. rettigeri, C. dweissus* and *P. mirabilis*. Intermediate activity was shown against *S. boydii,* and *S. sonnet* whereas *E. coli, S. flaxineri, S. dysentarica* and *S. pyogenes* were sensitive to this antibiotic. There was no action of chloramphenicol against *P. aeruginosa* and *P. mirabilis*. Slight activity was shown against *V. cholerae, S. typhi, S. typhimirium, S. boydii S. sonnei* and *C. dweissus*. Intermediate activity was shown against *P. rettigeri* whereas *E. coli, S. flaxineri, S. dysenterica* and *S. pyogenes* were sensitive.

For amikacin a slight activity was recorded for *V. cholerae and S. typhimrium*; intermediate activity was shown against *P. rettigeri, S. boydii, S. sonnei, S. dysenterica* and *C. dweissus*. *E. coli, P. aeruginosa, S. typhi, S. flaxineri, S. pyogenes* and *P.*

mirabilis were sensitive to this antibiotic. Cephalosporin showed no action against *S. flaxineri*. Slight action was shown against S. typhi, P. rettigeri, S. boydii, S. sonnei *and P. mirabilis.* Intermediate action was shown against *E. coli, C. dweissus*, and *S. pyogenes. P. aeruginosa, V. cholerae, S. typhimirium* and *S. dysenterica* were sensitive to this antibiotic.

Gentamycin showed slight activity against S. *typhimirium* and intermediate activity against *P. aeruginosa, V. cholerae, S. typhi, P. rettigeri, S. boydii, S. sonnei, C. dweissus, S. pyogenes* and *P. mirabilis*. Sensitivity was shown against *E. coli, S. flaxiner* and *S. dysenterica, E coli* was slightly affected by ampicillin. Intermediate action was shown by cephalosporin while it was sensitive to the rest of the antibiotics.

P. aeruginosa was resistant to cotrimoxazole. kanamycin and chloramphenicol. There was a slight activity against this micro-organism by ampicillin and tetracycline. The intermediate response was shown by gentamycin whereas amikacin and cephalosporin showed strong activity against this micro-organism.

V. cholerae was resistant to cotrimoxazole. Slight activity against this micro-organism was shown by ampicillin, tetracycline, kanamycin amikacin and chloramphenicol. The intermediate activity was shown by gentamycin whereas cephalosporin showed strong antimicrobial activity against this micro-organism.

S. *typhi* was resistant to tetracycline. Slight activity against this pathogen was shown by ampicillin, cotrimoxazole, kanamycin, chloramphenicol and cephalosporin. The intermediate activity was shown by gentamycin. Amikacin showed strong activity against this micro-organism. Slight activity against S. *typhimurium* was shown by ampicillin, tetracycline, cotrimoxazole, kanamycin, chloramphenicol, amikacin and gentamycin. Cephalosporin showed strong action against this pathogen.

P. rettigeri was resistant to ampicillin and was slightly affected by tetracycline, cotrimoxazole, kanamycin and cephalosporin. Intermediate action was shown by chloramphenicol, amikacin and gentamycin. S. flaxineri was resistant to ampicillin, cotrimoxazole and cephalosporin. It was slightly afiected by tetracyclin

strongly affected by kanamycin, chloramphenicol, amikacin and gentamycin.

S. boydii was resistant to tetracycline. It was slightly affected by ampicillin, chloramphenicol and cephalosporin. There was an intermediate reaction to kalam, amikacin and gentamycin. Cotrimoxazole strongly affected this micro-organism. *S. sonnei* was slightly affected by ampicillin, tetracycline, chloramphenicol and cephalosporin. It showed an intermediate response to cotrimoxazole, kanamycin amikacin and gentamycin.

S. dysenterica was slightly affected by ampicillin and tetracycline. It showed an intermediate response to amikacin but it was strongly affected by cotrimoxazole, kanamycin, chloramphenicol cephalosporin and gentamycin. *C. dweisus* was slightly affected by ampicillin, tetracycline, cotrimoxazole and kanamycin. It showed an intermediate response to amikacin, cephalosporin and gentamycin.

S. pyogenes was resistant to ampicillin but it showed intermediate response to cephalosporin and gentamycin. It was strongly affected by tetracycline, cotrimoxazole, kanamycin, chloramphenicol and amikacin. *P. mirabilis* Was resistant to cotrimoxazole and chloramphenicol. It was slightly affected by ampicillin, tetracycline, kanamycin and cephalosporin. It showed an intermediate response to gentamycin and was strongly affected by amikacin.

From Table 6 it can be seen that S. *pyogenes* and *P. aeruginosa* were the most and least sensitive micro-organisms respectively. This result was statistically significant at ($F12 \ 83=3.2$, $P<0.001$). *S. pyogenes* was the most inhibited while *P. aeruginosa* was the least inhibited micro-organism respectively. This result was statistically significant at ($F7, 83=2.94$, $P<0.001$).

(iii) Zones of inhibition (in mm) of ether, methanol and water-dipped and dried discs used in the extraction of plant parts of *Euphorbia hirta L.* tested against stock culture

The results summarized in Table 7 show that the negative controls had no inhibitory effects on microorganisms tested against them. The zones of inhibition are 6 mm for each micro-organism. This was the diameter of the disc. This implies that the solvents did not affect the micro-organisms tested against them.

(iv) Inhibition zone (in mm) for plant parts (roots, stems, leaves and flowers) of *Euphorbia hirta* L. tested against stock cultures

The results of the above tests showing the range of the size of the zone of inhibition for the individual plant parts are summarized in Table 8. The ether and water extracts showed low inhibitory growth effects on the stock cultures that they were tested against. The zone of inhibition by the root extracts is ether ranging from 6.1 mm to 11.1 mm. For the methanol extracts the range was from 6.3 mm to 12.1 mm and for the water extracts it ranged from 6.2 mm to 9.1 mm.

For the stem extracts the range was from 6.1 mm to 8.1 mm in the ether extracts, 7.2 mm to 9.1 mm in the methanol extracts and from 6.1 mm to 8.1 mm in the water extracts. In the leaf extracts the range of inhibition was from 6.1 mm to 8.1 mm in the water extracts. In the flower extracts, the range of inhibition was from 6.1 mm to 9.1 mm in the ether extracts 6.1 mm to 9.1 mm and from 7.1 mm to 12 mm in the water extracts.

(v) Zones of inhibition (in mm) of medicinal plants tested against local cultures

The results of the above tests are summarized in Table 9. The results show that *C. albicans* was resistant to the extracts of *A. aspera* whereas the rest of the micro-organisms from the stock cultures this extract showed slight activity. *A. conyzoides* extracts showed slight activity against seven of the eight local cultures that they were tested against and an intermediate activity against *S. aureus*. *B. grantii* extracts did not show any action against *C. albicans* but had slight action against all the rest of the stock cultures. *B. pilosa* extracts showed slight activity on all the stock cultures except *P. vulgaris* on which it showed intermediate activity. The extracts of *C. didymobotrya Dicrocephalum integrifolia, C. vitellimum, E. hirta, H. fuscus, L. camara, P. guajava, S. cainefolia, S. incanurn* and *T. mimuta* showed slight activity on all the stock cultures that they were tested against. *C. occidentalis* extracts showed slight activity against all the cultures that they were tested against except C. albicans on which it had no action.

T. brachyceras extract had slight activity on five of the stock cultures that they were tested against but showed intermediate activity on *B. subtilis, E. aerogenes* and *P. vulgaris, V. auriculifera* extracts showed slight activity against five of the stock cultures that they were tested against but they showed intermediate activity against *S. faecalis, B. subtilis,* and *E. aerogenes* and. *R. vulgaris* extracts showed slight activity against seven of the stock cultures that they were tested against but had no action on *C. albicans*.

B. pilosa, C. didymobotrya, E. hirta L., H. fuscus, P. guajava, S. cuinefolia, S. incanum, and *V. auriculifera* extracts showed slight activity on *C. albicans*. The range of inhibition for this fungus was from 6.1 mm to 11 mm.

A. aspera extract had an inhibition range of 7 min to 9 mm for seven of the micro-organisms it was tested against and it showed slight activity against all the seven bacterial species that it was tested against. *A. conyzoides* extract had an inhibition range of 7 mm. to 15 mm for all the micro-organisms tested against it. It showed slight activity against six bacterial species and the one fungus that it was tested against. The intermediate activity was shown against *S. aureus*. *B. grantii* showed an inhibition range of 7 mm to 9 mm for all the organisms tested against. *C. albicans* was resistant to this extract. *Bidens pilosa* had an inhibition range of 7.1 mm to 13 mm. The extract had slight activity on all the micro-organisms that it was tested against except *P. vulgaris* on which it had intermediate activity. The most sensitive micro-organism to this plant extract was *P. vulgaris* an inhibition zone of 13 mm.

C. occidentalis had a range of inhibition measuring from 7 mm to 8 mm. *C. albicans* was resistant to this extract. *C. vitellinum* extracts slightly affected all the microorganisms that they were tested against. *D. integrifolia* showed slight activity against six of the stock cultures that it was tested against but it showed intermediate activity on *S. faecalis* and *B. subtilis* The range of inhibition was from 7.1 mm. to 14 mm. i.e. from the highest to the lowest.

As for *E. hirta* the range of inhibition was from 7 mm to 10 mm. This extract showed slight activity on all the stock cultures that it was tested against. *H. fuscus* had a range of inhibition of 6.1 mm to 10 mm from the least sensitive to the most sensitive micro-organisms. This extract showed slight activity on all the stock cultures. For *Indigofera arrecta* the range of inhibition was from 7 mm to 9 mm. This extract showed slight activity on all the seven bacterial stock cultures that it was tested against. *C. albicans* was resistant to this extract. For *L. camara* the range of inhibition measured from 8.1 mm to 10 mm. This extract showed slight activity on all the stock cultures that it was tested against. For *O. basilicum* the range of inhibition measured 6.1 mm to 14 mm. This extract showed slight activity on seven of the stock cultures that it was tested against but intermediate activity on *P. vulgaris*.

P. guajava's range of inhibition was from 7 mm to 9 mm. This extract showed slight activity on all the stock cultures that it was tested against. For *R. vulgaris* range of inhibition was measured from 7 mm to 9 mm i.e. from least to most sensitive micro-organisms. *C. albicans* was resistant to this extract. *S. cuinefolia* had an inhibition range of 7 mm to 9 mm. This extract showed slight activity on all the stock cultures that it was tested against. *S. incamum*'s zone of inhibition measured 6.1 mm to 11 mm. This extract showed slight activity on all the stock cultures that it was tested against.

T. mimuta had a range of inhibition of 7.1 mm for the least sensitive micro-organism to 9.1 mm for the most sensitive micro-organism. This extract showed slight activity on all the stock cultures that it was tested against. *T. brachycerus*'s range of inhibition was from 6.1 mm to 13 mm i.e. from the least sensitive micro-organism to the most sensitive micro-organism. This extract showed slight activity on five of the stock cultures that it was tested against but had intermediate activity against *B. subtilis, E. aerogenes* and *P. vulgaris, V. auriculifera* had a range of inhibition measuring 7.1 to 13 mm. This extract showed slight activity against five of the stock cultures that it was tested against but intermediate activity against *S. faecalis*, *B. subtilis* and *E. aerogenes*.

(vi) Zones of inhibition (in mm) of medicinal plant extracts tested against clinical isolates and reference cultures from Kenyatta National Hospital

The results on the effects of the plant extract on clinical isolates are summarized in Table 10. Extracts of *A. aspera* showed slight activity on all the clinical isolates that they were tested against. *A. conyzoides* extracts showed slight activity on eleven of the clinical isolates. *S. faxineri* and *S. boydii* were resistant to these extract. *B. grantii* leaf extracts showed slight activity against ten clinical isolates but intermediate activity against *V. cholera* (Ogagwa) and *S. sonnei*. *P. rettigeri* was resistant to this extract.

B. pilosa leaf extracts showed slight activity against ten clinical isolates but intermediate activity against *V. cholerae* (Ogagwa), *S. typhimurium and S. sonnei*. *C. didymobotrya* leaf extracts showed slight activity against twelve clinical isolates but intermediate activity against *V. cholerae* (Ogagwa). *C. occidentalis* leaf extracts showed slight activity against eleven clinical isolates. *S. boydii* was resistant to this extract. *C. vitellinum* extracts showed slight activity against twelve clinical isolates but intermediate activity against *V. cholera* (Ogagwa).

D. integrifolia extracts showed slight activity against twelve clinical isolates but intermediate activity against *S. typhimurium*. *E. hirta* extracts showed slight activity against six, intermediate activity against two and sensitivity against four clinical isolates. *H. fuscus* extracts showed slight activity against ten isolates, intermediate activity against one isolate and sensitivity against one isolate. *P. aeruginosa* was resistant to this extract. *I arrecta* leaf extracts showed slight activity on four isolates but no action on the other nine activities on *V. cholerae* (Ogagwa) *O. basilicum* extracts showed slight activity on eight isolates and sensitivity to two. Three isolates were resistant to this extract. *P. guaiava* leaf extracts showed slight activity against eight isolates and intermediate activity against the isolates. *R. vulgaris* extracts were slightly active against twelve isolates. *S. dysenterica* was resistant to these extracts.

S. cuinefolia extracts were slightly active against eight isolates and showed intermediate activity to one isolate and sensitivity to one isolate. Three isolates were resistant to these extracts. *S. incanum* extracts showed slight activity against eight isolates and intermediate activity against three isolates. Two isolates were resistant to these plant extracts. *T. brachyceras* extracts were slightly active against eleven isolates but showed intermediate activity against two isolates.

T. minuta leaf extracts showed slight activity against twelve isolates and intermediate activity against one isolate. *V. auriculifera* extracts showed slight activity against twelve isolates but intermediate activity against one isolate. *O. basilicum* extract and *C. occidentalis* extract were the most and least inhibitory extracts respectively which were statistically significant at (F19, 228= 2.9, P< 0.001). *V.cholerae* (ogagwa) and S. typhi microorganisms were the most and least sensitive micro-organisms. The results were statistically significant at (F12, 218=3.2, P< 0.001)

B. pilosa, C. didymobotrya, E. hirta L., H. fuscus, P. guajava, S. cuinefolia, S. incanum, and *V. auriculifera* extracts showed slight activity on *C. albicans*. The range of inhibition for this fungus was from 6.1 mm to 11 mm.

A. aspera extract had an inhibition range of 7 mm to 9 mm for seven of the microorganisms it was tested against and it showed slight activity against all the seven bacterial species that it was tested against. *A. conyzoides* extract had an inhibition range of 7 mm. to 15 mm. for all the microorganisms tested against it. It showed slight activity against six bacterial species and the one fungus that it was tested against. The intermediate activity was shown against *S. aureus. B. grantii* showed an inhibition range of 7 mm. to 9 mm for all the organisms tested against. *C. Albicans* was resistant to this extract. *Bidens pilosa* had an inhibition range of 7.1 mm to 13 mm. The extract had slight activity on all the microorganisms that it was tested against except P. vulgaris on which it had intermediate activity. The most sensitive microorganism to this plant extract was *P. vulgaris* with an inhibition zone of 13 mm.

C. occidentalis had a range of inhibition measuring from 7 mm to 8 mm. *C. albicans* was resistant to this extract. *C. vitellinum* extracts slightly affected all the microorganisms that they were tested against. *D. integrifolia* showed slight activity against six of the stock cultures that it was tested against but it showed intermediate activity on *S. faecalis* and *B. subtilis*. The range of inhibition was from 7.1 mm. to 14 mm i.e. from the highest to the lowest.

As for *E. hirta* the range of inhibition was from 7 mm to 10 mm. This extract showed slight activity on all the stock cultures that it was tested against. *H. fuscus* had a range of inhibition of 6.1 mm to 10 mm from the least sensitive to the most sensitive micro-organism. This extract showed slight activity on all the stock cultures.' For *Indigofera arrecta* the range of inhibition was from 7 mm to 9. mm. This extract showed slight activity on all the seven bacterial stock cultures that it was tested against. *C. albicans* was resistant to this extract. For *L. camara* the range of inhibition measured from 8.1 mm to 10 mm. This extract showed slight activity on all the stock cultures that it was tested against. For *O. basilicum* the range of inhibition measured 6.1 mm to 14 mm. This extract showed slight activity on seven of the stock cultures that it was tested against but intermediate activity on *P. vulgaris*.

P. guajava's range of inhibition was from 7 mm to 9 mm. This extract showed slight activity on all the stock cultures that it was tested against. For *R. vulgaris* range of inhibition was measured from 7 mm to 9 mm i.e. from least to most sensitive micro-organisms. *C. albicans* was resistant to this extract. *S. cuinefolia* had an inhibition range of 7mm to 9 mm. This extract showed slight activity on all the stock cultures that it was tested against. *S. incanum*'s zone of inhibition measured 6.1 mm to 11 mm. This extract showed slight activity on all the stock cultures that it was tested against.

T. minuta had a range of inhibition of 7.1 mm for the least sensitive micro-organism to 9.1 mm for the most sensitive micro-organism. This extract showed slight activity on all the stock cultures that it was tested against. *T. brachycerus*'s range of inhibition was from.

TABLE 5

Zones of inhibition (in mm) of antibiotics tested against stock cultures

MICRO-ORGANISMS	ANTIBIOTICS							
	Amp	Tet	Cot	Kan	Chl	Amik	Ceph	Gen
S. faecalis	6.0	23.1±0.2	20.3±0.1	22.1±0.2	23.1±0.1	29.2±0.2	9.1±0.1	19.1±0.3
E. coli	6.0	16±0.1	22.1±0.2	20.2±0.2	21.2±0.1	19.1±0.2	6.1±0.2	19.1±0.2
P. aeruginosa	6.0	6.0	6.1±0.3	6.1±0.1	6.0	19.1±0.2	7.1±0.3	16.1±0.2
S. aureus	6.1±0.3	25±0.3	20.3±0.1	24.2±0.2	27.1±0.2	26.2±0.2	27.1±0.2	26.1±0.3
B. subtilis	16.1±0.3	24.1±0.3	6.0	17.2±0.1	24.1±0.1	22.1±0.1	21.1±0.3	25.1±0.1
E. aerogenes	6.1±0.2	25.1±0.3	22.1±0.3	27.1±0.1	6.1±0.1	18.1±0.3	9.1±0.1	8.1±0.2
P. vulgaris	6.1±0.2	6.1±0.1	6.1±0.2	18.1±0.3	6.1±0.2	19.1±0.2	15.1±0.1	15.1±0.2
C. albicans	21.1±0.1	11±0.2	23.1±0.2	20.1±0.2	27.1±0.3	26.1±0.3	27.1±0.2	27.1±

LEGEND:

S. faecalis: Streptococcus faecalis   B. subtilis =Bacillus subtilis

E. coli: Escherichia coli

E. aergenes: Enierobacter aerogenes

P. aeruginosa =Pseudomonas aeruginosa

P. vulgaris =Proteus vulgaris

S. aureus =SIreptococcus aureus

C. albicans: Candida albicans

Statistics = Two-way ANOVA with replication

Standard deviation=+

Amp=Ampicillin

Tet=Tetracyclille

Ceph=Cephalosporin.

Cot=Cotrimoxazole

Kan=Kanamycin.

Gen=Gentamycin.

Ch1=Chl0raphenical

Amik= Amikacin.

TABLE 6

Zones of inhibition (in mm) of reference antibiotics tested against clinical isolates and reference cultures

MICRO-ORGANISMS	ANTIBIOTICS							
	Amp	Tet	Cot	Kan	Chl	Amik	Ceph	Gen
E. coli	6.1±0.2	19.1±0.1	19.1±0.1	19.1±0.2	23.1±0.3	21±0.1	13.5±0.2	21.5±0.1
P. aeruginosa	6.1±0.2	6.1±0.1	6.0	6.0	6.0	18.1±0.3	18.1±0.1	13±0.2
V. cholera	6.1±0.3	6.1±0.2	6.0	8±0.2	10.1±0.2	6.1±0.2	18.1±0.1	14±0.3
E. typhi	7±0.3	6.0	7±0.2	9.1±0.1	7.1±0.1	18±0.4	8±0.1	15.1±0.2
S. typhimurium	6.1±0.2	7±0.2	8.1±0.1	8±0.2	8.1±0.1	8±0.2	20.1±0.2	7.1±0.3
P. rettigeri	6.0	6.1±0.2	6.1±0.1	7±0.3	13±0.1	15±0.2	6.1±0.2	13±0.2
S. flaxineri	6.0	6.1±0.2	6.0	18±0.1	22.1±0.2	21.1±0.2	6.0	22±0.3
S. boydii	6.1±0.2	6.0	19±0.2	17±0.2	6.1±0.1	15±0.2	6.1±0.3	14±0.1
S. sonnei	7.1±0.3	7.1±0.2	14.1±0.2	14.1±0.1	6.1±0.3	14.1±0.1	6.1±0.2	13.1±0.2
S. dysentarya	7.1±0.1	7.1±0.2	21.1±0.1	18±0.2	27.1±0.2	17.1±0.1	18.1±0.1	25±0.2
C. dweisus	8.1±0.2	8±0.3	9±0.2	8.1±0.1	11±0.3	17±0.1	16±0.3	15.1±0.1
S. pyogenes	6.0	24±0.3	24.1±0.1	22.1±0.2	22.1±0.2	23±0.2	17.1±0.1	17.1±0.2
P. mirabilis	6.1±0.2	6.1±0.2	6.1	9.1±0.1	6.0	18.1±0.2	8.1	16.3

LEGEND:

E. coli=Escherichia coli: P. aeruginosa=Pseudomonas aeruginosa; V. cholera: Vibrio cholera(ogagwa};

S. typhi=Salmonella typhi; S. typhimurium=Salmonella typhimurium; P. rettigeri: Proteus rettigeri; P. mirabilis =Proteus mirabilis; S. flaxineri: Shigella flaxineri; S. boydii=Shigella boydii; S. sonnei

sonnei; S. dysentarya=Shigella dysentarya; C. dweisus=Citrobacter dweisus; S. pyogenes=Streptococcus pyogenes

Statistics: Two-way ANOVA with replication;

Standard deviation=+

TABLE 7

Zones of inhibition (in mm) of solvents treated and dried used in the extraction of plant parts

| MICRO-ORGANISMS | SOLVENTS | | |
	Ether	Methanol	Water
E. coli	6.0	6.0	6.0
P. aeruginosa	6.0	6.0	6.0
V. cholera (ogagwa)	6.0	6.0	6.0
S. typhi	6.0	6.0	6.0
S. typhimurium	6.0	6.0	6.0
P. rettigeri	6.0	6.0	6.0
P. mirabilis	6.0	6.0	6.0
S. flaxineri	6.0	6.0	6.0
S. boydii	6.0	6.0	6.0
S. sonnei	6.0	6.0	6.0
S. dysenterica	6.0	6.0	6.0
C. dweisus	6.0	6.0	6.0
S. pyogenes	6.0	6.0	6.0

LEGEND.

E. coli=Escherichia coli: P. aeruginosa=Pseudomonas aeruginosa; V. cholera: Vibrio cholera(ogagwa};

S. typhi=Salmonella typhi; S. typhimurium=Salmonella typhimurium; P. rettigeri: Proteus rettigeri; P. mirabilis=Proteus mirabilis; S. flaxineri: Shigella flaxineri; S. boydii=Shigella boydii; S. sonnei

sonnei; S. dysenterica=Shigella dysenterica; C. dweisus=Citrobacter dweisus; S. pyogenes=Streptococcus pyogenes

TABLE 8

Inhibition zones (in mm) for plant parts (roots, stems, leaves and flowers) of E. hirta L. tested against local culture

MICOR-ORGANISMS	Stems E M W	Leaves E M W	Roots E M W	Flowers E M W
S. faecalis	7.2+0.1	7.2+0.2	7.1+0.1	6.1+0.2
	8.2+0.2	11.1+0.1	10.1+0.2	8.1+0.2
	8.1+0.1	7.2+0.2	.1+0.1	7.1+0.1
E. coli	6.2+0.2	7.2+0.2	6.1+0.2	7.2+0.1
	8.2+0.3	9.5+0.1	9.1+0.1	8.1+0.3
	6.1+0.4	1+0.1	7.1+0.1	7.1+0.1
P. aeruginosa	7.1+0.3	8.1+0.1	7.2+0.3	7.2+0.2
	8.1+0.2	9.2+2.7	7.1+0.2	6.1+0.2
	7.1+0.1	7.1+0.1	7.1+0.1	7.1+0.1
S. aureus	8.1+0.3	9.1+0.2	8.2+0.1	6.4+0.2
	8.3+0.2	9.3+0.2	7.2+0.2	10.1+0.2
	7.2+0.2	6.2+0.3	8.2+0.3	7.1+0.1
B. subtilis	6.1+0.2	8.2+0.1	7.1+0.2	6.1+0.3
	7.1+0.2	9.1+0.3	8.1+0.1	9.1+0.1
	6.1+0.3	7+0.2	7.1+0.3	7.1+0.1
E. aerogenes	7.1+0.1	6.1+0.2	11.1+0.1	9.1+0.1
	9.1+0.2	8.1+0.2	12.1+0.2	14.2+0.2
	7.1+0.1	6.1+0.3	6.2+0.1	7.1+0.1
P. vulgaris	7.1+0.2	7.2+0.2	6.2+0.2	7.1+0.1
	7.1+0.3	8.1+0.4	6.3+0.2	9.2+0.2
	7.1+0.2	7.1+0.1	6.2+0.1	12.1+0.1
C. albicans	8.1+0.1	8.1+0.2	7.1+0.2	9.1+0.2
	8.1+0.1	8.1+0.1	9.1+0.3	11.2+0.3
	8.1+0.1	8.1+0.3	9.1+0.1	7.1+0.1

LEGEND

E= ether extract   M= Methanol extract   W= Water extract

S. faecalis = *Streptococcus faecalism; E. coli=Escherichia coli; P. aeruginosa=Pseudomonas aeruginosa; S. aureus= Streptococcus aureus; B. subtilis= Bacillus subtilis; E. aerogenes=Enterobacter aerogenes; P. vulgaris=Proteus vulgaris; C. albicans=Candida albicans*

Statistics: Two-way ANOVA with replication

Standard deviation: +

TABLE 9

Zones of inhibition (in mm) of plant extracts of the medicinal plants tested against local cultures

MICRO-ORGANISMS	PLANT EXTRACTS									
	Aa	Ac	Bg	Bp	Cd	Co	Cv	Di	Eh	Hf
S. faecalis	8±0.1	9±0.2	7±0.3	8.2±0.4	9±0.2	8±0.2	8±0.1	14±0.3	8±0.1	10±0.2
E. coli	8±0.2	8±0.3	7±0.2	8.1±0.1	9±0.2	8±0.4	7±0.2	7.1±0.1	8.1±0.2	10±0.3
P. aeruginosa	7±0.1	8±0.1	7±0.4	8.1±0.2	8±0.1	7±0.2	8±0.1	7.1±0.1	7.1±0.3	9.1±0.1
S. aureus	7±0.2	15±0.2	8±0.1	10±0.3	9±0.1	7±0.2	8±0.1	10±0.1	7.1±0.1	9.1±0.2
B. subtilis	8±0.1	8±0.1	9±0.3	7±0.2	9±0.1	8±0.3	9±0.1	13±0.2	8±0.2	8.1±0.1
E. aerogenes	8±0.2	7±0.1	8±0.3	9.1±0.1	8±0.2	8±0.1	9±0.1	9.7±0.2	7.1±0.1	8.1±0.1
P. vulgaris	9±0.3	7±0.3	7±0.1	13±0.2	7±0.1	8±0.3	8±0.2	8.4±0.1	7±0.2	9.1±0.1
C. albicans	6.0	9±0.1	6.0	7±0.1	8±0.2	6.0	8±0.1	7.1±0.3	10±0.1	6.1±0.1

LEGEND:

Abbreviations used in Table 9 for the selected medicinal plants

Aa=Achryanthes aspera; Ac=Ageratum conyzoides; Bg=Bidens grantii; Bp=Bidens pilosa; Cd=Cassia didymobotrya; Co=Cassia occidentalis; Cv=Crassocephalum vitellinum Di=Dicrocephalum integrifolia; Eh-Euphorbia hirta; Hf=Hibiscus fuscus

TABLE 9 Contd.

Zones of inhibition (in mm) of plant extracts of the medicinal plants tested against local cultures

PLANTS EXTRACTS

MICRO-OR-GANISMS	La	Lc	Ob	Pg	Rv	Sc	Si	Tb	Tm	Va
S. faecalis	7±0.1	10±0.2	11±0.1	8±0.2	8±0.1	8±0.2	11±0.1	10±0.1	9.1±0.2	12±0.1
E. coli	8±0.2	9.1±0.1	11±0.2	9±0.1	8±0.1	8±0.1	9.1±0.2	10±0.1	9.1±0.1	10±0.2
P. aeruginosa	9±0.1	9.1±0.1	7.1±0.1	9±0.1	7±0.1	7±0.2	9.1±0.1	11±0.1	8.1±0.1	11±0.1
S. aureus	6.0	8.1±0.1	7.1±0.2	7±0.1	8±0.1	7±0.1	8±0.2	11±0.1	9.1±0.1	7.1±0.1
B. subtilis	7±0.1	8.1±0.1	6.1±0.2	7±0.2	9±0.1	8±0.3	8.1±0.1	12±0.1	7.1±0.1	13±0.3
E. aerogenes	7±0.1	8.1±0.2	6.1±0.1	7±0.1	7±0.2	7±0.1	7.1±0.1	13±0.1	7.1±0.1	12±0.1
P. vulgaris	8±0.1	9.1±0.2	14±0.1	8±0.2	8±0.1	7±0.2	7.1±0.1	12±0.1	7.1±0.1	9.1±0.1
C. albicans	6.0	9.1±0.1	11±0.1	7±0.2	6.0	9±0.1	6.1±0.1	6.1±0.2	11±0.1	9.1±0.1

LEGEND

Ia=Indigofera arrecta; Lc=Lantana camara; Ob=Ocimum basilicum; Pg=Psidium guajava; Rv=Rhus vulgaris; Sc=Sida cuinefolia; Si=Solamum incanum; Tb=triumfetta brachyceras; Tm=Tagetes minuta; Va=Varmonia auriculifera

TABLE 10

Zones of inhibition (in mm) of extracts of plants tested against clinical isolates and reference cultures

MICRO-ORGANISMS	PLANT EXTRACTS									
	Aa	Ac	Bg	Bp	Cd	Co	Cv	Di	Eh	Hf
E. coli	6.1±0.2	6.1±0.3	10.1±0.1	8.1±0.1	11±0.1	6.1±0.1	10±0.2	6.1±0.2	12±0.1	6.1±0.2
P. aeruginosa	6.1±0.2	6.1±0.1	6.1±0.3	11±0.2	7.1±0.2	6.1±0.2	7.1±0.3	13±0.3	7.1±0.2	6±0.2
V. cholera	6.1±0.2	6.1±0.2	14.1±0.2	13±0.1	12±0.2	6.1±0.2	12±0.2	11±0.2	27±0.1	31±0.1
S. typhimurium	9.1±0.1	6.1±0.1	9.1±0.2	17±0.2	9.1±0.2	6.1±0.2	8.1±0.2	13±0.4	9.1±0.3	6.1±0.2
P. rettigeri	7.1±0.2	6.1±0.2	6.0	9.1±0.1	6.1±0.1	6.1±0.1	8.1±0.2	9.1±0.2	8.1±0.2	6.1±0.4
P. mirabilis	6.1±0.2	6.1±0.4	6.1±0.2	9±0.3	6.1±0.2	6.1±0.3	7.1±0.2	10±0.4	20±0.1	6.1±0.1
S. flaxineri	6.1±0.3	6.0	6.1±0.4	9.1±0.1	7.1±0.3	6.1±0.2	7.1±0.2	10±0.1	16±0.1	6.1±0.3
S. boydii	6.1±0.2	6.0	6.1±0.2	8.1±0.2	9.1±0.1	6.0	9±0.2	7±0.4	18±0.1	6.1±0.1
S. sonnei	7.1±0.1	6.1±0.2	12±0.1	14±0.1	11±0.1	6.1±0.2	8.1±	6.1±0.2	19±0.2	6.1±0.2
S. dysenterica	7±0.2	6.1±0.1	6.1±0.1	9.1±0.2	7±0.2	6.1±0.1	8.1±0.2	10±0.3	28±0.3	13±0.1
C. dweisus	7.1±0.2	6.1±0.2	9.1±0.2	8.1±0.1	9±0.4	6.1±0.2	7.1±0.2	9.1±0.1	6.1±0.2	11±0.2
S. pyogenes	6.1±0.4	6.1±0.3	7.7±0.1	11±0.2	7±0.2	6.1±0.1	7.1±0.4	9.1±0.2	8.1±0.4	6.1±0.3
S. typhi	6.1±0.1	6.1±0.2	8.1±0.2	9.1±0.1	7.1±0.2	6.1±0.4	9.1±0.2	8.1±0.2	6.1±0.1	6.1±0.2

LEGEND

Aa=Achryanthes aspera; Ac=Ageratum conyzoides; Bg=Bidens grantii; Bp=Bidens pilosa; Cd=Cassia didymobotrya; Co=Cassia occidentalis; Cv=Crassocephalum vitellinum; Di=Dicrocephalum integrifolia Eh=Euphorbia hirta; Hf=Hibiscus fuscus

TABLE 10 Contd

Zones of inhibition (in mm) of extracts of plants tested against clinical isolates and reference cultures

MICRO-ORGANISMS	PLANT EXTRACTS									
	La	Lc	Ob	Pg	Rv	Sc	Si	Tb	Tm	Va
E. coli ATCC 25922	6.0	6.1± 0.2	6.1+0.3	10± 0.1	8+0.1	6.1+0.2	6.0	7± 0.2	11± 0.4	7.8± 0.2
P. aeruginosa ATCC28783	6.0	6.1± 0.4	6.1±0.2	6.1± 0.2	8+0.2	8±0.2	6.1± 0.2	7.2± 0.2	7.1± 0.2	6.8± 0.2
V. cholera (Ogagwa) KO17	6.0	15± 0.1	31+0.2	16± 0.1	6.1±0.2	28±0.3	6.1± 0.4	9.1± 0.2	13± 0.2	14± 0.2
S. typhymirium KO12	6.0	6.1± 0.4	6.1+0.1	10± 0.2	11±0.2	6.0	6.0	13± 0.2	8.1± 0.3	8.7± 0.1
P. rettigeri KO39	6.0	6.1± 0.1	6.1+0.3	12± 0.1	7.1±0.3	6.1±0.2	6.1± 0.2	9.1± 0.1	8± 0.11	7.2± 0.4
P. mirabilis KO09	6.0	6.1± 0.1	6.1±0.2	11± 0.1	7.1±0.1	6.1±0.2	6.1± 0.1	11± 0.1	7.1± 0.2	8± 0.2
S. flaxineri KO08	6.0	6.1± 0.2	6+0.2	15± 0.1	7.1±0.4	6.1±0.2	11± 0.1	9.1± 0.2	7.1± 0.3	8± 0.2

Organism	Ia	Tm	Lc	Ob	Pg	Rv	Sc	Si	Tb	Va
S. boydii K032	8 ± 0.1	8.1 ± 0.3	6.0	10 ± 0.4	7.1 ± 0.1	6.1 ± 0.2	12 ± 0.2	6.1 ± 0.2	9 ± 0.1	8.3 ± 0.1
S. sonnei K032	8 ± 0.1	6.1 ± 0.2	30 ± 0.1	15 ± 0.2	8.1 ± 0.4	6.1 ± 0.1	13 ± 0.2	10 ± 0.3	8 ± 0.4	10 ± 0.3
S. dysentoria K018	8 ± 0.2	11 ± 0.2	6.1 ± 0.2	14 ± 0.2	6.0	7.1 ± 0.1	14 ± 0.2	8.1 ± 0.3	8 ± 0.2	9.5 ± 0.2
C. dweisus K006	6.0	6.1 ± 1	6.1 ± 0.3	8.1 ± 0.2	6.1 ± 0.2	6.0	6.1 ± 0.3	7.1 ± 0.2	7.1 ± 0.1	7.3 ± 0.2
S. pyogenes ATCC 581899	6.0	14 ± 0.3	6 ± 0.4	8.1 ± 0.1	8.1 ± 0.2	14 ± 0.2	7.1 ± 0.2	12 ± 0.2	7.1 ± 0.1	8.2 ± 0.1
S. typhi K060	8 ± 0.1	7.1 ± 0.1	8.1 ± 0.2	9.1 ± 0.2	7.1 ± 0.4	7.1 ± 0.4	7 ± 0.2	9.1 ± 0.1	9.1 ± 0.1	7.7 ± 0.2

LEGEND

Ia=Indigofera arrecta; Tm: Tagetes minuta Lc= Lantana camara; Ob=Ocimum basilicum; Pg: Psidium guajava; Rv: Rhus vulgaris; Sc=Sida cuinefolia; Si =Solanum incanum; Tb=Triumfetta brachyceras; Va=Vernonia auriculifera.

Chapter Five

Phytochemical Screening

5.1 Materials and Methods

The present procedure for the phytochemical screening of the plant extracts was the one described by Chhabra et al. (1984) (Figure 2). Following this procedure, the qualitative presence of certain phytoconstituents can be detected with much certainty. A schematic flow diagram of the method employed for the screening is shown in Figure 2.

10-15 g of the powdered plant material was repeatedly extracted with ether (3 x 50 ml.) (Stage 1) at room temperature, with shaking at intervals of 1 hour. The resulting solutions were filtered using Whatman filter paper No. 1. The solvent from the combined ether extracts was distilled off and the residue dissolved in ethanol (30-40 ml.) and then divided into two portions. A portion of the extract (1.1) was tested for the presence of alkaloidal bases and volatile oils while the other portion of the extract (1.2) was saponified with alcoholic potassium hydroxide (10 ml., 0.5 N) by refluxing in a water bath for 1 - 2 hours. The alcohol was distilled off and the residue was redissolved in hot distilled water (10-15ml). The non-saponifiables (1.21) were extracted with ether (3x10ml) and tested for the presence of carotenoids, and steroids/triterpenoids.

The alkaline aqueous solution (1.2) Was acidified with concentrated hydrochloric acid pH 3-4) and extracted with ether (3x 15 ml.). This ethereal solution (1.22) was tested for the presence of coumarins, emodins, fatty acids and flavonoids.

The plant material, Mac (a), after repeated extraction with ether, was repeatedly extracted with hot methanol (3 x 50 ml.) (Stage 2). The combined extracts Were concentrated under reduced pressure to one-third of their original volume and divided into two portions. To a portion of the extract (2.1) chemical reactions were performed for the detection of alkaloidal salts, reducing compounds and tannins while the other portion (2.2) was hydrolyzed with hydrochloric acid (10 ml., 10%) by refluxing on a water bath for 30 min. the contents were cooled and distilled water added (15 ml.) and extracted with ether (3xx10 ml) The ether extract (2.21) was tested for the presence of anthracenes, coumarins, flavonoids and steroids/triterpenoids while the acidic aqueous solution (2.22) was tested for the presence of anthocyanins.

Mac (b) after repeated extraction with ether and methanol was repeatedly extracted with hot water (3 x 50 ml) (Stage 3-Mac.c). The combined water extracts were concentrated under reduced pressure to one-third of their original volume and divided into two portions. To a portion of the water extract (3.1) chemical reactions were performed for the presence of alkaloidal salts, polyuronoids, reducing compounds, saponins, starch and tannins. The other portion (3.2) was hydrolyzed with hydrochloric acid and screened as hydrolyzed methanol extract (2.2). 3.2 is treated in the same manner as 2.2

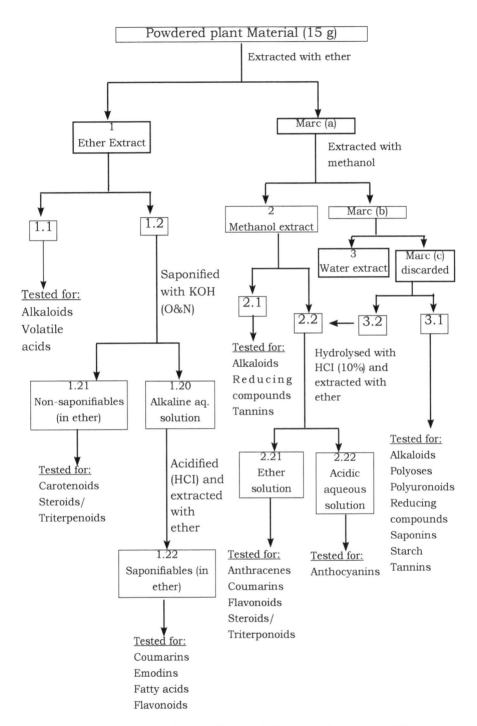

FIGURE 2: Schematic outline of the method used for phytochemical screening

Performance of specific tests

Each of the tests for individual classes of compounds was performed using about 5 ml. of the individual plant extract. The specific tests used were those described by Chhabra et al. (1984).

(i) Alkaloids

Alkaloids were tested in all three extracts, ether, methanol and water. In the ether extract; ether solution (1.1) was evaporated and the residue macerated with hydrochloric acid (2%, 1.5 ml). The resulting acidic solution was divided into three parts. To one part was added Mayer's reagent and to another Wagner's reagent while the third acted as a blank. In the alcoholic extract, methanol solution (2.1) was evaporated and the residue macerated with hydrochloric acid (2%, 1.5 ml.), filtered, basified with ammonium hydroxide (10%) and extracted with ether. The ether-soluble portion was evaporated,

dissolved in hydrochloric acid (2%, 1.5 ml), divided into three parts and tested as in the ether extract (1.1).

In the Water extract, aqueous solution (3.1) was basified with ammonium hydroxide (10%) and extracted with ether (3 x 10ml). The ether solution was dissolved with hydrochloric acid (10%) and the acidic aqueous solution was divided into three parts and tested as in the ether extract (1.1) i.e. to one part add Mayer's reagent and another Wagner's reagent while the third acted as a blank.

A+ reaction was recorded upon the production of faint turbidity by either one or both reagents. A++ was recorded if a light opalescence precipitate was observed and a +++ reaction was recorded if a heavy yellowish-white precipitate was observed.

(ii) Anthocyanins

Methanol and water extracts were tested for anthocyanins. The appearance of red colour at pH 3-4 and the change of colour with pH modification (pH 8-9) in the acidic aqueous solution (2.22) of methanol and water extract of (3.22) indicated the presence of anthocyanins.

(iii) Anthracene glycosides

The Water and methanol extracts were tested for anthracene glycosides. The appearance of a red colour by the addition of ammonium hydroxide (25%) to a portion of the ether solution (2.21), of methanol extract and ether solution (3.21) of the water extracts (indicated the presence of anthracene glycosides.)

(iv) Carotenoids

Only the ether solution (1.1) was tested for carotenoids. 10 ml of the extract was evaporated to dryness and a saturated solution of antimony trichloride in chloroform (2-3 drops) was added (Carr Price's reaction). In addition to concentrated sulphuric acid, carotenoid pigments first tum blue and later become red.

(v) Emodin (polyketide)

A portion of the ether solution (1.22) Was evaporated and the residue dissolved in benzene. If on the addition of ammonium hydroxide (25%), a red colour appeared, the presence of emodin was concluded.

(vi) Flavonoids

Flavonoids were tested for in all three extracts. The ether solution (1.22) and (2.21) of methanol and (3.21) of water extracts were evaporated to dryness. The residue was dissolved in methanol (50%, 1-2ml) by heating, then magnesium metal and concentrated hydrochloric acid (1-2 ml) was added. A red or orange colour indicated the presence of flavonoids.

(vii) Polyoses

Only the water extract was tested for polyose. The appearance of red colour by the addition of a few drops of concentrated sulphuric acid and alcoholic thymol to a portion of the evaporated extract (3.1) indicated the presence of polyose.

(viii) Starch

Only the water (3.1) extract Was tested for starch. The appearance of a blue colour by the addition of Lugol solution in the Water extract indicated the presence of starch.

(ix) Steroids/triterpenoids

All three extracts, ether, methanol and water were tested for steroids and triterpenoids. The ether solution (1.21) and the water and methanol solutions (2.21) were tested (Libermann-Burchard's reaction), 10 ml of each extract was evaporated to dryness and the residue dissolved in 0.5 ml of acetic anhydride followed by the addition of 0.5 ml. of chloroform. The solution was transferred to a dry test tube and 1.2 ml. of concentrated sulphuric acid was added from the side of the tube. A brownish-red or violet ring at the contact zone with a green or violet supernatant denoted the presence of steroids/triterpenes. A + reaction was recorded in tests for anthocyanins, anthracene glycosides, carotenoids, emodins, flavonoids, polyses, starch and steroids/triterpenoids when a slight colouration was observed, a ++ reaction was recorded when a medium intensity colouration was observed; and a +++ reaction was recorded when a strong colouration was observed.

(x) Coumarins

All three extracts, ether, methanol and Water were tested for coumarins. The ether solutions (1.22) and (2.21) of methanol and (3.21) water extracts were evaporated and dissolved in a small amount of hot distilled water. UV fluorescence at (=254nm of these aqueous solutions and the increase in intensity after the addition of ammonium hydroxide (10%) indicated the presence of coumarins.

When a slight fluorescence was observed, this was recorded as a +. A ++ reaction was recorded for medium fluorescence and a +++ reaction for a strong fluorescence.

(ix) Fatty acids

Only the ether extract was tested for fatty acids. A portion of the ether solution (1.22) was evaporated on a piece of filter paper and the transparency was noted. A + reaction was recorded when slight transparency Was observed, a ++ reaction was recorded when medium transparency was observed, and a +++ reaction when a strong fluorescence was observed.

(xii) Polyuronoids

The water extract (3.1) was tested for polyuronoids. A portion of the extract was mixed with an equal volume of haemotoxylin solution. The formation of a persistent violet precipitate insoluble in ethanol indicated the presence of polyuronoids.

(xiii) Reducing compounds

Methanol (2.1) and water extracts (3.1) were tested for reducing compounds. To a portion of the extracts (2.1) and 3.1) a few drops of Fehling's solution (A and B) were added. The appearance of a red precipitate on heating the mixture indicated the presence of reducing compounds.

(xiv) Tannins

Tannins were tested in the methanol and water extracts (2.1) and (3.1) by the gelatin-salt block test. Methanol and Water extracts (2.1) and (3.1) were separately divided into three parts. A sodium chloride solution was added to one portion of each test extract, 1% gelatin solution to each second portion and the gelatin-salt reagent to each third portion. Precipitation with the latter reagent, or with both the gelatin and gelatin-salt reagents was indicative of the presence of tannins.

Precipitation with the salt solution (control) indicated a false-positive test. Positive tests were further confirmed by the addition of a few drops of dilute ferric chloride to the test extracts, which gave a blue-black/green-black colouration. A + reaction was recorded in tests for polyuronoids, reducing compounds and tannins when a slight precipitate was observed; a ++ reaction when a medium precipitate was observed and a +++ reaction when a heavy precipitate was observed.

(xv) Saponins

The presence of saponins was tested in the Water extract. The honeycomb froth in a portion of the water extract (3.1) persists after shaking for 10 seconds, and a positive Liberian-Burchard reaction in the hydrolyzed solution (2.21) indicated the presence of saponins. A + sign was indicated when the froth reached a height of 0.5cm, a ++ sign with a height of up to 1cm, and a +++ sign with a height of more than 1cm.

(xvi) Volatile oils.

Volatile oils were tested in the ether extract. An aromatic smell in the evaporated ether extract (1.1) indicated the presence of volatile oils. A + sign indicated a slight aromatic smell, a +++ sign indicated a moderate aromatic smell and a +++ sign indicated a strong aromatic smell.

5.2 Results

The results are summarized in Table 11. The screening covered mainly nitrogenous compounds, acetogenins, polyketides, isoprenoids and carbohydrates.

Screening for nitrogenous compounds was mainly concerned with alkaloids whereas acetogenins and polyketides covered mainly tannins, flavonoids, coumarins, emodin, anthocyanins, anthracene glycosides and fatty acids. Twelve plant samples (60%) gave a positive reaction to alkaloids, and fourteen plant extracts (70%) tested positive for tannins. Twelve plants (60%) tested positive for flavonoids. Seventeen plants (85%) gave a positive test for coumarins. Five plants (25%) showed the presence of anthocyanins. Seven plants (35%) tested positive for anthracene glycosides, six plants (30%) showed the presence of fatty acids and nine plants (45%) tested positive for emodin.

Screening for isoprenoids was confined to steroids/triterpenoids, saponins, volatile oils and carotenoids whereas that for carbohydrates included polyuronoids, polyoses, reducing compounds and starch. Seventeen plants (85%) tested positive for steroids/triterpenoids, thirteen plants (65%) showed the presence of saponins, seventeen plants (85%) tested positive for volatile oils while ten plants (50%) showed the presence of carotenoids. Nine plant samples (45%) showed the presence of polyuronoids. Eleven plant samples (55%) tested positive for polyoses, 18 plants (90 %) positively tested for reducing compounds while two plant samples (10%) showed a positive reaction for starch.

TABLE 11

Phytochemical screening of the twenty selected medicinal plants E=Ether extract; M=Methanol extract; W=Water extract

Plant name	Part used	Alkaloids			Anthocyanins		Anthracene glycosides		Carotenoids
		E	M	W	M	W	M	W	E
A. Aspera	Stem	+	+	+	-	-	-	-	-
A. conyzoides	Leaf	-	-	-	-	-	-	-	+
B. grantii	Leaf	-	-	-	-	-	-	-	-
B. pilosa	Leaf	-	-	-	-	-	-	-	+
C. didymobotrya	Leaf	++	++	++	++	++	++	-	
C. occidentalis	Leaf	-	-	-	-	-	-	-	-
C. vitellinum	Flower	-	-	-	-	-	++	-	-
D. integrifolia	Plant	-	--	-	-	-	-	-	++
E. hirta	Plant	++	+++	+	++	++	++	++	+
H. fuscus	Leaf	+	+	-	-	-	-	-	-
I. arrecta	Leaf	-	-	-	-	-	-	-	-
L. camara	Leaf	-	-	-	+	+	-	-	+
O. basilicum	Leaf	-	-	-	-	-	-	-	-
P. guajava	Leaf	-	-	-	-	-	-	-	+
R. vulgaris	Leaf	-	-	-	++	+++	+	++	+
S. cuinefolia	Leaf	++	++	-	-	-	-	-	-
S. incanum	Leaf	+	++	-	-	-	-	-	+
T. minuta	Leaf	-	-	-	-	-	-	+	+
T brachycerus	Leaf	-	-	-	+	-	+	-	+
V auriculifera	Leaf	-	-	-	-	-	++	-	-

TABLE 11 Contd

Screening of the twenty selected medicinal plants E=Ether extract; M=Methanol extract; W=Water extract

Plant name	Part used	Emodins	Flavonoids			Polyoses	Starch
		E	E	M	W	W	W

A. Aspera	Stem	-	-	-	-	-	-
A. conyzoi-des	Leaf	+	+	+	+	-	-
B. grantii	Leaf	-	+	+	+	-	-
B. pilosa	Leaf	+	+	+	+	-	-
C. didymo-botrya	Leaf	++	-	-	-	-	-
C occidentalis	Leaf	+	-	-	-	+	-
C. vitellinum	Flow-er	-	-	-	+	++	-
D. integrifolia	Plant	-	-	-	-	++	-
E. hirta	Plant	++	++	++	++	+	-
H. fuscus	Leaf	-	-	-	+	-	-
I. arrecta	Leaf	-	+	+	-	++	++
L. camara	Leaf	-	-	-	-	+	-
O. basilicum	Leaf	-	++	++	++	+	-
P. guajava	Leaf	-	-	+	-	++	-
R. vulgaris	Leaf	-	+	++	++	++	-
S. cuinefolia	Leaf	-	-	-	-	-	-
S. incanum	Leaf	+	-	-	-	+	-
T. minuta	Leaf	-	+	+	-	-	-
T brachyc-erus	Leaf	-	-	-	-	-	-
V auriculifera	Leaf	+	+	+	+	++	+

TABLE 11 Contd

Screening of the twenty selected medicinal plants listed in Table 3
E=Ether extract; M=Methanol extract; W=Water extract

Plant name	Part used	Compounds tested for							
		Steroids/ triter-penoids			Coumarins			Fatty acids	Polyur-onoids
		E	M	W	E	M	W	E	W
A. Aspera	Stem	+	+	+	+	+	+	+	+
A. conyzoides	Leaf	-	+	+	++	++	++	+	+
B. grantii	Leaf	+	++	++	-	-	-	-	+
B. pilosa	Leaf	-	-	-	+	+	+	-	-
C. didymo-botrya	Leaf	-	-	-	+	+	+	-	+

C. occidentalis	Leaf	-	-	-	+	+	+	-	-
C. vitellinum	Flower	+	+	+	-	-	+	-	++
D. integrifolia	Plant	+	+	+	-	-	++	-	++
E. hirta	Plant	++	++	-	+	++	+++	++	+
H. fuscus	Leaf	++	-	-	+	+	+	-	-
I. arrecta	Leaf	+	++	-	++	++	+	+	-
L. camara	Leaf	-	+	-	+	+	+	+	-
O. basilicum	Leaf	+	+	++	+	+	+	-	-
P. guajava	Leaf	+	+	+	-	++	-	+	-
R. vulgaris	Leaf	++	+++	+++	+	+	+	-	-
S. cuinefolia	Leaf	++	++	+	+	+	+	-	-
S. incanum	Leaf	+	+	+	+	+	+	-	+
T. minuta	Leaf	-	+	-	+	+	+	-	-
T brachycerus	Leaf	-	+	-	O+	+	+	-	-
V auriculifera	Leaf	+	++	+	-	+	+	-	+

TABLE 11 Contd

Screening of the twenty selected medicinal plants E=Ether extract; M=Methanol extract; W=Water extract

		Compounds tested for					
		Reducing compounds		Tannins		Saponins	Volatile Oils
Name of plant	**Part used**	M	W	M	W	W	W / E
A. Aspera	Stem	-	++	-	-	+	-
A. conyzoides	Leaf	-	-	+	+	+	+
B. grantii	Leaf	++	++	++	-	+	+
B. pilosa	Leaf	+	++	+	+	-	+
C. didymobotrya	Leaf	+	+	+	+	-	+
C. occidentalis	Leaf	++	++	+++	++	-	-
C. vitellinum	Flower	++	-	+	+	++	+
D. integrifolia	Plant	-	++	+	++	+	+
E. hirta	Plant	-	-	+++	+	+	+
H. fuscus	Leaf	+	+	++	-	+	-
I. arrecta	Leaf	++	++	-	-	-	+

L. camara	Leaf	++	+	++	++	+	+
O. basilicum	Leaf	+	++	-	-	+	+
P. guajava	Leaf	-	++	+++	+++	+	+
R. vulgaris	Leaf	-	++	++	++	-	+
S. cuinefolia	Leaf	+	+	-	-	+	+
S. incanum	Leaf	+++	+++	-	-	+	+
T. minuta	Leaf	++	++	-	-	-	+
T brachycerus	Leaf	++	+	++	-	+	+
V auriculifera	Leaf	++	-	+	+	++	+

Chapter Six

Discussion

6.1 Ethnomedical Aspects

6.1.1 Traditional Medicine and Medicinal Plants

From the taxonomic consideration of the medicinal plant drugs, the Thallophyta were represented by the Agricaceae and the Pteridophyta by the Aspleniaceae. The rest of the plant drugs came from the Spermatophyta. Five families namely the Graminae, and the Palmae, represented the Monocotyledonae, the Liliaceae the Dioscoreaceae and the Zingiberaceae. The rest of the medicinal plants were from the Dicotyledoneae.

This study revealed that the Abagusii indeed possess an extensive knowledge of the effective medicinal properties of their flora. One hundred and sixty-six plant species representing 138 genera and 62 families were botanically identified. It was also revealed that medicinal plants supply medication to the vast majority of people in both urban and rural areas. This information was obtained from the interviews with the traditional healers who knew the backgrounds of their patients well. Some medicinal plants have been in use since time immemorial but through the ages, by trial and error, many plants have gained fame as healing agents and some of these have fingered on as is in the case of *Euphorbia hirta*.

In this ethnic group, it was found that there is a great variety of healing practices for, example, steam inhalation techniques, fumigations like incense, bloodletting, hydrotherapy and many other beliefs Most of the traditional healers do not distinguish between the physical and psychological elements of an illness and thus largely rely on.

In this group, medicinal plants are components of a medical system, rather than the sole medicinal resource; animal products, mineral substances and certain other methods are also used. Common plant treatments are known and used by the majority of rural people in addition to those used by traditional specialist healers.

There is no distinction between what is consumed as food or medicine. Some medicinal plants such as *Ipomea batatas, Solanum nigrum, manihot esculenta*, and *Gynandra gynandopsis*, to mention just a few, are consumed as vegetables in this ethnic community and also by other Kenyan communities (Maundu et al, 1999; Ogol et al, 2002). Foods are thought to have different healing qualities and plants are often added to foods or are taken as tonics to promote good health. It should be noted that plant medicines can contribute important minerals and vitamins to the diet, thus favouring overall health e.g. the small fruits of *Rhus vulgaris* which are edible contain vitamin C which prevents scurvy. This finding is in agreement with the results of Sheng-ji (1989) who found out that the traditional cultures of ethnic groups in Northwest China use flowers as food materials and medicines. The Abagusii also use flowers as food and medicine.

From the literature it was found out that most studies on traditional medicine do not assess plant material as it is traditionally prepared e.g. in conjunction with other plant materials nor do they examine the extent to which treatments are used. No studies attempt to place a value on the health care provided by traditional healers and traditional plant medicines in terms of the costs of their modern equivalents. Thus While there is a vast amount of literature (Johansson et al., 1987; Johansson & Alakoski-Johansson, 1988; Lindsay, 1978; Morgan, 1980; Morgan, 1981; Timberlake, 1987; Tanaka, 1983; Barrett, 1996; Kokwaro. 1993; Watt & Breyer-Brandwijk, 1962) on which species have been or are currently used in traditional medical treatments, there is little information to assess their effectiveness.

6.1.2 Plant Resources Used as Medicines

Thus, although botanic studies have identified a vast array of medicinal plants in Eastern and Southern Africa (Johansson et al. 1987; Johansson & Alakoski-Johansson, 1988; Lindsay, 1978; Morgan, 1980; Morgan; 1981; Timberlake, 1987; Tanaka, 1983; Barrett, 1996; Kokwaro, 1993; Watt & Breyer—Brandwijk, 1962) which have been or are currently used in traditional medical treatments there is little information to assess their effectiveness. It is also difficult to distinguish between past and present medicinal uses of these plants. This makes it difficult to evaluate the extent to which plant resources are currently used as medicines and to identify the most important species that will need urgent conservation measures.

6.1.3 Studies of Plant Medicines Used by Specific Groups

While local studies have been undertaken (Johansson et 21., 1987; Johansson & Alakoski-Johansson, 1988; Lindsay, 1978; Morgan, 1980; Morgan, 1981; Timberlake, 1987; Tanaka, 1983; Barrett, 1996; Kokwaro, 1993; Watt & Breyer—Brandjwik, 1962) illustrating the breadth and variety of species which are exploited over a region, in-depth household studies which would provide more information on how and when different species are used are lacking regarding this group.

The Abagusii classify sickness as "simple" (treatable by family members or with Western medicine). The different types of ailments are associated with particular plant treatment, for example, diseases of the intestines, problems specific to women and the health of the newborns, improvement of the quality of milk in lactating women, fungal infections, bacterial infections etc., are treated using particular plants. Simple illnesses such as stomachaches, toothaches, diarrhea, etc. are normally treated in the family. Many treatments involve a combination of plants.

Many households as was revealed by the healers, continuously use plant medicines. The people generally distinguish between those plant species or remedies common to all or used by all the people and those known only or restricted to specialized healers. Women were found to be generally knowledgeable regarding common medicines and they usually manage the collection, preparation and administration of the medicines. Generally, they learn about plant medicines from their mothers. This is particularly true concerning young mothers during their first pregnancy when there is much to be said for the rule of never giving any medication without traditional medical advice. The sound rule is for the young mother to heed all the advice she is given during her first pregnancy from the traditional birth attendant's clinic and from her mother. With this and a modicum of common sense, she should have little difficulty in coping with the minor elements of her first born. As her family grows, so does her skill. Other specialists (generally men) on the other hand undergo long apprentice periods learning about different plant treatments.

Although traditional health systems are thought to rely principally on curative rather than preventative practices, it was found that many household treatments are both preventative and curative. Mothers generally administered herbal cures to prevent diseases such as dysentery, diarrhea etc., especially to young children. Plants are also taken as general tonics, either in infusions, decoctions or baths. For primary dental care, sticks made from stems, bark or roots of different species are chewed several times daily to clean and freshen teeth and they were found to be popular in both urban and rural areas.

6.1.4 The Extent to which the Abagusii Use Medicinal Plants

Information on the general popularity of plant medicines among the Abagusii was lacking and there is no way in which such information can be deduced from this kind of study unless the traditional healing practices inherent in this group are assessed. Such information and the information on the extent to which the people themselves as opposed to being provided by traditional healers use medicinal plants would make a very interesting topic for research.

However, it was noted that most of the Abagusii are increasingly shifting to the use of plant medicines and this could be attributed to the fact that Western medicines are very expensive due to the rising cost of drugs and the negative experiences (or disillusion) with modern drugs and the modern health care system that has been experienced by these people. In this group, traditional cures are often used before turning to Western medicine and *vice versa*. The majority of people prefer herbal medicine because it is familiar (tradition and experience) and less expensive than antibiotics in pharmacies and markets.

6.1.5 The Effectiveness of Plant Medicines

From the literature, it was noted that most studies, which address the effectiveness of different traditional medical treatments generally evaluate their potential for pharmaceutical development, thus information can only be found in chemical and pharmacological studies, that analyze the phytochemistry of different species. However, the majority of these studies generally present their results in terms of a plant's chemical composition. They don't link the presence of a particular compound in a plant e.g. tannins with the use of the plant in traditional medicine. They rarely examine the combined effects of many plant treatments. In addition, the potential health benefit(s) that plant minerals provide are not considered. Thus the layman is at a loss to judge the effectiveness of a particular plant for treating a particular illness or as one element of the complete traditional healing system.

Since plants contain a multiplicity of constituents, it has been often claimed that the use of the whole plant or many whole plants rather than one purified constituent may be more effective therapeutically and also produce fewer adverse effects (Wright and Phillipson, 1990). This observation could support the practice whereby traditional healers mostly prefer to use more than one plant in the preparation of their medicines and also the reason why, if one plant is used in one treatment, then another must be taken as well to eliminate the toxic effect of the first plant.

The results revealed that the healers use different plant species from the same family to treat the same disease condition(s). This observation is supported by the work of other researchers. In their work, Parr *et al.* (1990) analyzed 1000 individual plants of the genera *Datura, Scopolia* and *Hyoscyamus* to establish the variations in the levels and patterns of tropane alkaloids that occur between plants. These results showed that there were substantial differences observed between alkaloid patterns between different species, but the qualitative differences observed between different lines were less than those shown between plants.

During this study, an attempt was made to link the antimicrobial activity and the presence of a particular compound, for example, flavonoids to the use of a particular plant in traditional medicine. The results obtained demonstrated that the plants that have traditionally been used in treatments (especially bacterial and fungal infections) contained chemical constituents, which could explain or justify their effectiveness in traditional medical treatments. However, it should be noted that not all traditional medicines have proven effective in the scientific sense of the word.

6.1.6 The Availability of Plant Medicine Resources

Traditionally plant medicines used to be gathered from forest areas, fallow lands, village common lands as well as agricultural fields. This study revealed that plant species usually used by traditional healers come from specific locations, which may be very far from the villages. During this study, one healer remarked that the availability of plant medicines was seasonal and that they were often very rare during the dry season and plentiful during the rains. He also observed that often the medicinal effectiveness of a plant is thought to be highest from plants collected in the Wild and particular areas. Plant medicines collected from deep in the forest are thought to be stronger medicinally. This observation is in agreement with the finding that the medicinal qualities of *Euphorbia hirta* L. are stronger when gathered from the wild rather than from cultivated areas and that they contain higher concentrations of active constituents in the wild (ENDA, 1987). This finding is also in agreement with the work of

Mizuo *et al.* (1990) who in their studies in the estimation of the quality of *Epidium* leaves as a crude drug by the examination of the content of flavanol glycosides by high liquid performance chromatography in nineteen species collected from different parts of the world, Europe, China and Japan, found that the species from Japan and China had abundant quantities of flavonal glycosides when compared to the European ones. This also supports the fact that sometimes the healers would send for a plant that they use in their medicinal preparations from a different geographical region. For example, a traditional healer might send for a specimen of *E. hirta* L. from the Coast Region while the same species is available locally in the Nyanza region. Even within the same region, there could be ecological or even micro-ecological differences.

An important observation that was made in this study concerns the rapid disappearance of many indigenous herbal medicinal plants with some such as *Gloriosa superba* L. being virtually on the verge of extinction. Some of the signs of the disappearance of these medicinal plants could be seen from the observation that people walk long distances to collect them and that some medicinal plants are no longer found. Areas that used to be thick forests of diverse species of flora have been reduced to bushland and are now fast disappearing. It was also noticed that many medicinal plants are not maturing and seeding because young plants are being harvested before they mature and the number of traditional healers using herbs is also falling.

Some of the factors responsible for this disappearance of herbal medicinal plants are that the rising numbers of people and animals cause pressure on plant survival. Natural habitats are being cleared for farming and grazing and trees are felled for timber, charcoal and other commercial uses. The pattern of land use has also changed. The land is grabbed and used in ways that are not sustainable.

Inappropriate ways of harvesting, for example, the removal of all the bark or uprooting the whole plant without leaving any part to grow, bush fires, commercialization of plant resources, lack of awareness that plants are the sources of conventional medicine, young people not interested in practicing traditional medicine, the view by some western religions that the use of traditional medicine is a form of evil worship or witchcraft and the poverty in the area that makes people to fell trees and cut them for sale to earn a livelihood are also contributory factors to the disappearance of the medicinal plants.

6.2 Chemical and Biological Studies: A Comparative Analysis

The results summarized in Table 8 show that the leaf extracts have high inhibitory effects (F_{11}, 77=3.2, p<0.001). Herein might lie the explanation as to why the leaves are preferred in the treatment of thrush, diarrhea and dysentery in small children. It should also be remembered that the whole plant is preferred in such treatments. The results summarized in Table 8 also show that all the plant parts have inhibitory effects on all of the pathogenic micro-organisms that they were tested against whereas the results of the chemical analysis summarized in Table 11 reveal that all the plant parts contain compounds such as alkaloids, anthocyanins, anthracene glycosides, carotenoids, coumarins, emodins, flavonoids, saponins, steroids/triterpenoids, tannins and volatile oils, all known to be of medicinal value (Trease & Evans, 1978).

The root, stem, leaf and flower extracts of ether, methanol and water inhibited the growth of all the micro-organisms that they were tested against. This justifies the use of the whole plant in traditional medicine in the treatment of thrush, diarrhea and dysentery. However, the leaves are mostly preferred. The results summarized in Table 8 and Table 11 support the reason Why most traditional healers prefer to use the leaves most of the time. The dry powdered leaf extract of the whole plant is burned into ash, made into a tisane and administered orally for the treatment of acute diarrhea which is a bacterial disease brought about by toxin-producing bacteria such as *V. cholerae, E. coli,*

Shigella spp, *Staphylococcus aureus* and *Salmonella* spp. The results of this investigation clearly showed that all the plant parts inhibited the growth of E. coli and S. aureus which are toxin-producing bacteria-associated diarrhea diseases. Acute diarrhea is a major killer of children under seven years in this community.

It is also significant to note the most sensitive organism to these extracts was *Candida albicans* (F7, 77=17.7, P< 0.001), a fungal pathogen and the leaf and root were the most and least inhibitory plant extracts respectfully (F3, 77=5.9, P<0.001). *C. albicans* and *P. vulgaris* were the most and least sensitive micro-organisms (F77,17=2.7, P<0.001).

Individual parts of the plant did not show any significance concerning the extraction solvent (F2, 3=3.2, P<0.001). Methanol seems to be the most efficient when the effectiveness of the extraction solvents is compared. The result is statistically significant at (F2, 3=3.2, P< 0.01). This may be because methanol is an intermediate solvent able to extract both polar and non-polar compounds.

Out of the sixteen compounds screened for phytochemicals, methanol was involved in the extraction of eight compounds, which was half of the compounds screened for and water was involved in the extraction of eleven compounds. Methanol was second to water as an extraction solvent. This fact should be noted because water is the solvent commonly used as an extraction solvent in traditional medicine.

The active principles seem to come out more in the intermediate methanol extract and the water extract, a strong polar solvent. Most traditional remedies are prepared in the form of powders, saps, poultices, baths, decoctions in local gin, water, concoctions, infusions and teas. Decoctions and infusions in water are the most popular forms of preparations. In this study, it Was revealed that most traditional healers prepared their medicinal plant potions as aqueous extracts. Other traditional healers prepare their medicinal potions in the form of tinctures (alcohol extracts) although this method was found not to be popular with the majority of the healers. These results serve as a justification for the traditional use of all plant parts of *E. hirta* in the preparation of traditional herbal remedies used in treating some of the ailments afflicting this community.

The reason for this is that all the plant parts contain active therapeutic principles and the use of solvents such as water, local gin e. g. *busaa* (alcoholic extract) in the preparation of decoctions, tisanes, concoctions and infusions for the extraction of compounds of medicinal value from medicinal plants can also be justified on these grounds. The results also confirm the use of methanol as a good extracting solvent for the qualitative chemical determination of extracted compounds. The possibility that other unknown compounds of medicinal value can be extracted by less polar compounds such as diethyl ether should not be ruled out.

The results summarized in Table 5 show that *P. vulgaris*, which is known to cause wounds, responded to all the eight antibiotics that it was tested against. *P. aeruginosa* was not susceptible to three antibiotics namely ampicillin, tetracycline and chloramphenicol. *B. subtilis* was resistant to cotrimoxazole. The results summarized in Table 10 show that all the plant extracts of the medicinal plants inhibited the growth of all stock bacterial cultures. For P. vulgaris the most inhibitory effect was caused by the leaf extracts of *O. basilicum* (14.0 mm). These results clearly show that these plants could be good candidates for the treatment of diseases caused by these bacterial species. *C. albicans* was resistant to the extract of *A. aspera, B. grantii C. occidentalis, I. arrecta* and *R. vulgaris*.

The results summarized in Table 5 show that *S. faecalis, E. coli* and *P. auruginosa* were resistant to ampicillin. *S. faecalis* is known to cause a sore throat and *E. coli, P. auruginosa* and *S. aureus* are known to cause bacteria that cause wounds. These results would imply that ampicillin cannot treat the cause of the disease caused by bacteria. The results summarized in Table 6 also clearly show that the majority of the common antibiotics in the market such as gentamycin, amikacin and others are still effective in that they inhibited the growth of the majority of the bacterial species and the fungi. *C. albicans* that they were tested against. Their zones of inhibition were quite high in the majority of the microorganisms that they were tested against.

Results summarized in Table 9 show that all the bacteria species except *S. aureus* were susceptible to all twenty medicinal plant extracts. *S. aureus* was not susceptible to the extracts from *I. arrecta*. *C albicans* were not susceptible to the extracts of *A. aspera. B. grantii, C. occidentalis, I. arrecta,* and *R vulgaris.* The fact that these medicinal plant extracts inhibited the growth of these micro-organisms could imply that all these extracts have active principles of therapeutic value that could be used to combat various diseases such as wound infections that are caused by pathogenic bacteria such as *P. aeruginosa* and fungal infections such as ringworm. The results summarized in Table 9 also show that the majority of the microorganisms were susceptible to the medicinal plant extracts. These results demonstrate that all the twenty medicinal plants screened for antimicrobial activity could serve either individually or in combination as remedies in the treatment of diseases caused by the micro-organisms that they were tested against. In other words, these plants could substitute conventional antibiotics such as ampicillin and others in the treatment of infectious diseases brought about by bacterial and fungal agents.

The results of the tests using clinical isolates are summarized in Table 10. Nine clinical isolates were not susceptible to the extracts from *I. errecta E. coli* was not susceptible to the extracts of *I. arrecta* and *S. incanum. P. aeruginosa* was not susceptible to the extracts of *H. fuscus, I. arrecta* and *S. cuinefolia. V. cholera* (Ogagwa) was not susceptible to the extract from *I. arrecta. S. typhimurium* was not susceptible to *I. arrecta, S. cuinefolia* and *S. incanum. P. rettigeri* was not susceptible to the extracts of *B. grantii* and *I. arrecta. S. flaxineri* was not susceptible to the extracts from *A. conyzoides, I. arrecta* and *O. basilicum. S. boydii* was not susceptible to the extracts from *A. conyzoides* and *O. basilicum. C. dweissus* was not susceptible to the extracts from *I. arrecta* and *S. cuinefolia. S. pyogenes* was not susceptible to the extracts from *I. arrecta* and *O. basilicum.* These results are a clear demonstration that medicinal plants contain active principles that can hinder the growth and proliferation of several pathogenic micro-organisms that are of clinical significance thus making them potential candidates in the production of drugs that will be helpful in the fight against disease-causing pathogens. These results are in agreement with the findings of other researchers (Mitscher et al., 1987). This finding implies that there is a possibility for the development of new inexpensive drugs based on phytochemicals from plants. The galenicals, which are crude medicinal extracts, could then be processed in Kenya in the form of liquid extracts, tinctures, decoctions, dry extracts etc. Such drugs will be cheaper to prepare, acceptable, accessible and affordable to the majority of the people in the urban and rural areas. Herein, also lies the reason for the conservation of plants from different regions within the country.

Comparatively, seventeen of the plant extracts tested against *S. tyhimurium* hindered its growth. This result is in agreement with the observation that some difficult diseases such as eczema that conventional medicine cannot treat may be managed by traditional medicine (Sheehan et al., 1992; Braquet et al., 1991).

Nineteen of the twenty extracts tested against the clinical isolates inhibited the growth of *V. cholera* (Ogawa) the causative agent of the deadly cholera. This implies that even traditional healers using extracts of medicinal plants can treat cholera which is also treated by conventional medicine. This will lend credence to the idea that perhaps the greatest gain to be made in integrating traditional and orthodox systems of medicine into the official health care system of a developing nation is that the increase in manpower would help to provide total health coverage for all before 2010.

In the present study, it was revealed that plant extracts are effective in hindering the growth and proliferation of a wide range of pathogenic micro-organisms such as *S. typhimurium*, which is known to cause gastroenteritis often called food poisoning. This implies that such plant extracts are possible candidates in the fight against diseases caused by these micro-organisms.

In the phytochemical screening, it was found that the twenty plants that were screened contained different chemicals of medicinal value such as alkaloids, tannins, coumarins, etc. These observations reveal similar results in the past (Kubo & Taniguchi, 1988: Caceras *et al.*, 1993; Oligashi, *et al.* 1991; Okemo, 1996; Okemo & Mwatha, 2002) reveal that African plants, in particular medicinal plants, constitute a rich, but still largely untapped pool of natural products. These observations also support the hypothesis that the medicinal plants used by Abagusii traditional healers have therapeutic value and it is possible to develop cheap drugs from these renewable plant resources. At this juncture, a study on the standardization of herbal potions, dispensing them to patients in specified doses or strictly regulated quantities would be highly recommended.

Very recently *Ancistrocladus* alkaloids have even become candidates as possible drugs against the Immune Deficiency Syndrome AIDS - one of the great medical and social challenges of our time (Bringmann *et al.*, 1996). This implies that the plants which showed the presence of alkaloids are also possible candidates for the production of anti-malarial drugs and drugs against AIDS and that the incorporation of traditional medicine in primary health care programmes would be a cost-effective endeavour as proposed by the WHO (1972).

In the phytochemical screening a total of sixteen compounds were screened for and of these, ten Were secondary metabolites. Currently, the drugs produced by the pharmaceutical industries for the treatment of various human and livestock diseases are secondary metabolites of plant origin such as alkaloids, tannins, etc. It would be better to search for these compounds in various plant species using data collected from ethnomedical sources on the uses of various plants in the treatment of various disease conditions.

6.3 Seasonability and Chemical Constituents

The study also revealed that the Abagusii traditional healers took great exception to the time and even the season when they do their plant collections. For instance, the healers strongly recommend that E. *hirta* samples for medicinal preparations should be collected very early in the morning. This practice is supported by the work of other research workers who have shown that the active constituents of plants can vary in quantity and quality from season to season. This variation may only be slight in some cases but in others, it is quite significant. For example, it has been shown that apart from geographical variations observed in the constituents of *Piper guiniense* there is also a seasonal variation which is important when this plant is used in traditional medicine (Addae Mensah *et al.*, 1977). Greunweller *et al.* (1990), in their work, found out that the biological activities of furastanol saponins from *Nicotiana tabacum* accumulate during ripening and are degraded during the germination of the seeds. The saponins were not found in any part of the plant. This also supports the idea that in traditional medicine plant part to be collected is of paramount importance. This finding implies that the seeds must be harvested during the ripening time to have the desired medicinal value. This finding also underscores the importance of the morphological part of the plant to be collected. The saponins found in this plant showed hemolytic and fungicidal activity. The fact that the saponins showed fungi toxic activity during the bioassay would justify the use of this plant in the treatment of ringworm and other fungal infections.

There is also increasing evidence that the yield of some plant constituents can even vary within 24 hours, this generally being due to the interconversion of compounds (Trease & Evans 1978). This variation in the concentration of active constituents can also be explained by the phenomenon of carbon dioxide fixation by PEP carboxylase. It is well-known as part of crassulacean acid metabolism (CAM) and is characteristic of desert succulents (Ting, 1985). In CAM, carbon dioxide fixation occurs at night and carbon dioxide is released again in the daytime for photosynthesis. The malic acid produced by fixation is probably transported into the vacuole and the concentrations achieved would depress the cytoplasmic pH values to below 3 when this is shipped back and decarboxylated in daylight it is likely to lead to a decrease in cytoplasmic pH values (Luttge &

Smith, 1982). Such a decrease in pH values would also affect the concentration of the active principles in the plant. Hence, the reason why the season and even the time of harvesting of a medicinal plant is of crucial importance in the use of the plant in traditional medicine. Thus although the traditional healer is not aware of these scientific facts, at least he/she knows the best time when to collect his/her plant specimens for the optimum yield of the desired product.

The age of the plant during harvesting is also considered. For example, traditional healers usually collect young plants of *E. hirta* for use in their herbal preparations. This can be explained scientifically by the fact that the age of the plant when harvested may determine not only the total amount of active constituents but also the relative amounts of each component. Such a traditional practice is supported by the work of El-Said *et al.* (1969) who have shown that *Ocimum gratissimum* L. produces the most volatile oil per unit weight when young. This is because the number of oil-secreting hairs does not increase appreciably when the leaf increases in Weight. This implies that such a plant should be harvested in the early stages of development. This observation is also supported by the work of Sainsbury and Sofowora (1971) Who observed that although the relative composition of terpenoids in the volatile oil of *O. gratissimum* does not vary with age (Sainsbury & Sofowora, 1971), there are instances Where a marked change in volatile oil occurs. For example, the young plants of *Mentha piperita* L. yield mostly pulegone but this is replaced by menthone and menthol in mature plants (Trease & Evans, 1978). These observations are also supported by the Work of Penera *et al.* (1988) who found out that changes in the content of essential oils, flavonoids and santonin in the dry matter in some Solanaceae plants varied from 0-5% depending on rainfall before anthesis and the plant age. The highest percentage involvement of essential oil was observed in the inflorescences at the time of anthesis and lowest in the overground mass during the time of growth. The oil's composition changed along with plant development. The percentage involvement of flavonoids such as quercetin and its derivatives also varied along with plant development.

In the screening of *E. hirta* no quantitative determination of the active principles was done for each plant part individually. Most traditional healers prefer to use leaves in their herbal preparations. It would be an interesting topic for research to compare the relative amounts of compounds in the various plant parts. Why should these healers mostly prefer the leaves and not the roots, stems, or flowers?

During his collections, the traditional healer took into consideration the morphological part of the plants collected. This practice is supported by the findings of other research workers. For instance, it has been found that although all aerial parts of *Ocimum gratissimum* L. produce oils of similar composition, the leaf is the richest (3.2%-4.1%) while the stem contains only traces of oil (El-Said et al., 1969; Sainsbury & Sofowora, 1971). Therefore, the collection of the stem merely increases the bulk of plant material to be processed. For an optimal yield of an active product it has been found that leaves should generally be collected as the flowers are beginning to open, flowers just before they are fully expanded and underground organs such as roots or rhizomes as the aerial parts begin to wither and die (Trease & Evans, 1978)

Takeshi et al. (1990), in their study on flavonol glycosides and other constituents from the leaves of *Ampelopsis brevipedunculata* Trautv. using the method of the distribution of these glycosides in various parts of the plant found that in the leaves, the glycosides containing arabinose and galactose were the main components, while in the fruits, the glycosides containing glucose and rhamnose were the main components. The ratio of monoglycosides to diglucosides was found to be higher in the ripe fruit than in the young fruit. These findings also lend support to the importance of the morphological part and the age of the plant during collection. The practice of considering the age of the plant during collection is also supported by other findings elsewhere. For example, in West Africa traditional healers usually use boiled yellow old leaves of *Carica papaya* L.

to bathe children suffering from skin rashes. They specifically instruct their patients to use the dead leaves that have fallen off the tree rather than the green leaves still turgid and on the tree. There is experimental evidence to the effect that the dead leaves are usually brown and richer in phenolic constituents than the green leaves. Also, the plant would have passed into the dying leaves certain unwanted metabolites that may be those required for medicinal purposes (Sofowora, 1982).

The collection of the plant parts also followed a certain pattern. For optimum yield of an active product it has been found that the collection of plant parts should generally be collected in the following order: leaves when the flowers are beginning to open, flowers just before they are fully expanded and underground organs such as roots or rhizomes just as senescence of the aerial parts sets in (Trease & Evans, 1978). Aerial parts were not collected during wet conditions. The explanation given for this was that if a collection is done under such conditions then the collected material would decompose thus leading to mould attack during storage. The barks were collected after or during a rainy season or damp weather since they often peel off readily from the wood. Gummy material or exudates from trees were collected during dry weather when they were less difficult to handle. During the collections, the healers excluded unwanted matter, which would increase bulk and cause adulteration. For instance, during the collection of gums, plant debris was eliminated while roots and other underground organs were freed from the soil by Washing them with clean water or brushing. Each vegetable drug product was carefully examined for unwanted materials such as discoloured flowers or leaves diseased or spoiled from insect attack.

During this investigation, it was found that there was a relationship between the antimicrobial effects of the plant extracts, the phytochemistry of the plant and the use of each of the twenty plants in their use in traditional medicine by the Abagusii traditional medical practitioners.

The practice of collecting a plant at a particular time is in agreement with the observation made by Addae Mensah *et al.*

(1977) that the active principles of a plant can vary in quality and quantity from time to time and from season to season and that this variation may only be slight in some cases but in others, it is quite significant. In one study they found that apart from geographical variations observed in the constituents of *Piper guiniense* there was also a seasonal variation that is important when this plant is used in traditional medicine. There is also scientific evidence that the yield of some plant constituents can vary within 24 hours, this generally being due to the Interco version of compounds (Trease & Evans, 1978). Thus although the traditional healer is not aware of these scientific facts, at least he/she knows the best time when to collect his/her plant specimens for the optimum yield of the desired product.

It would be an interesting topic for a study to do a phytochemical analysis of plant extracts of *Euphorbia hirta* from plants of different ages because traditional medical practitioners consider the age of the plant during the time of collection. They usually collect young plants of *E. hirta* for use in their herbal preparations. This observation is also in agreement with other researchers. This result is supported by the results of El-Said *et al.* (1969) who showed that *Ocimum gratissimum* produces the most volatile oil per unit weight when young. They found out that the number of oil-secreting hairs does not increase appreciably when the leaf increases in weight. They, therefore, concluded that the age of the plant during harvesting may determine the total amount of active constituents and also the relative amounts of each component. Such a conclusion implies that the harvesting of such a plant should be done in the early stages of development. This observation is also in agreement with the work of Sainsbury and Sofowora (1971) who observed that although the relative composition of terpenoids in the volatile oil of *O. gratissimum* does not vary with age, there are instances where a marked change in volatile oil occurs, for example, the young plants of *Mentha piperita* yield mostly pulegone but this is replaced by menthone and menthol in mature plants (Trease & Evans, 1978).

6.4. Chemical Composition and Biological Activity

The results summarized in Table 9 and 10 show that the leaf extract of *O. basilicum* exhibited inhibitory effects on the growth of all the stock cultures and ten clinical isolates that they were tested against. *S. faecalis* and E. coli which are normal flora in most animals and anaerobic bacterial genera such as *Streptococcus* species which comprise most of the bulk of the microbial flora in the large intestine may sometimes become harmful to the host. This may be the reason why this plant is used in the treatment of stomach pains, and nasal and bronchial catarrh.

The results summarized in Table 11 show that the plant contains volatile oils, which are known for their repellant properties and their action of hindering the growth and proliferation of bacteria. From this, it can be concluded that this plant could be an effective remedy for Wound infections.

The results in Table 9 and Table 10 show that *S. occidentalis* (L) Link. inhibited the growth of all the bacterial stock cultures and twelve of the clinical isolates that it was tested against. It did not inhibit the growth of *S. boydii*.

The results of Table 11 show that *C. occidentalis* (L) Link contains emodin (a polyketide) which has been reported to have the anthraquinone nucleus which is known to have laxative or purgative properties (depending on the dosage). With a powerful effect, they act by stimulating peristaltic movement in the large intestines and thus diminishing water absorption. As a result, the transit of the faeces is quicker as they are less dry. This is enough reason to justify the use of this plant's traditional medicine as a purgative and the treatment of various bacterial infections.

The results of Table 9 and Table 10 show that the leaf extracts of *L. camara* L. show inhibitory effects on all the bacterial stock cultures and all the clinical isolates that it was tested against. *E. coli, E. aerogenes, P. aeruginosa, S. aureus* and *P. vulgaris* are well-known bacterial species that cause wounds. This would justify the use of this plant as a remedy for throat afflictions.

The inhibitory effects of the leaf extract of this plant in most bacterial species it was tested against would justify the use of this plant in the treatment of toothache. Toothache is usually brought about due to bacterial decay.

Results summarized in Table 11 show that *L. camara* contains tannins, which are well known for their astringent properties and, hence, their usefulness in the treatment of sore throat. The plant extract also contains saponins, which are usually terpene derivatives, which have the property of diminishing surface water tension, producing the formation of foam just like soap. In vitro, they provoke haemolysis (destruction of the red blood corpuscles). Hence their expectorant properties (making the mucous secretion more fluid), thus ensuring their expulsion; they also act as diuretics, healing agents and analgesics. The presence of saponins in this plant justifies its usefulness in the treatment of coughs.

The results of Table 9 and Table 10 show that the leaf extracts of *P. guajava* show inhibitory effects against all the stock cultures and the clinical isolates that they were tested against. *E. coli, S. aureus, V. cholerae, S. sonnei, S. boydii, S. flaxineri, S. typhimurium* and *S. typhi* all of which are well-known pathogens that cause diarrheal diseases and dysentery were also inhibited. Results from Table 11 show that the leaf extract of *P. guajava* tested positive for tannins, which are phenolic compounds that coagulate gelatin and other proteins. They have astringent, haemostatic, antiseptic and invigorating properties. Tannins dry the skin and mucosa, easing the resolution of inflammatory processes and thus helping in wound healing. Their astringent property i.e. constricting blood vessels (vasoconstriction) gives them the medicinal value of preventing and controlling hemorrhages. Guava is one of the richest fruits in vitamin C since some of their varieties have five times the amount present in oranges. The leaves and root bark of the guava tree are very rich in tannins. Hence its usefulness in the treatment of diarrhea and dysentery.

Another reason why this plant is used in traditional medicine in the treatment of acute diarrhea and dysentery lies in the fact that the plant contains essential oils (volatile oils) which are well known for their action in regulating intestinal movements, preventing and controlling violent contractions and thus aiding the orderly flow of the food through the bowels and thus calming an otherwise over-active gut. Volatile oils are also known for their anti-microbial activity (El-Said et al., 1969). Therefore, the anti-microbial effect of the extracted volatile oil is probably a sufficient explanation for the anti-microbial effect.

Psidium guajava L. is used as a cold infusion, as such extracts have the advantage of extracting other active ingredients of plants yet only a minimal amount of tannins. When taken in high doses, tannins may prevent the absorption of certain minerals such as calcium and iron, as well as vitamins. Therefore, continuous intake of plants rich in tannins for long periods (more than one month) is not recommended. Plants rich in tannins such as tea, *Thea sinensis* are not recommended for pregnant women because habitual consumption may lead to constipation, stomach acidity, insomnia and nervous excitation and finally addiction as with any drug. The practice of using cold extracts in traditional medical preparations by the work of El-Said et al., (1969) with *O. gratissimum.* found that if the crude vegetable drug of the plant was boiled to form a decoction it contained less volatile oils than the cold infusion. It was also found that such aqueous decoctions were devoid of anti-microbial activity than the cold infusion but they do relax the guinea pig ileum and rat jejunum in vitro. Such decoctions could, therefore, still be effective in calming an overactive gut and thus curing diarrhea. Volatile oils are steam volatile.

Traditionally, a plant like *O. gratissimum* is also used to stop bleeding wounds and nose infections. The chemical analysis of its oil reveals that it has anti-bacterial activities similar to other antibiotics, and is especially effective against Salmonella spp. and E. coli, which causes sinusitis (Anyiwo, 1986).

Volatile oils can also act as demulcents and emollients. This alone is justification for the use of *P. guajava* L. in the treatment of diarrheal diseases and dysentery, which are both diseases of bacterial origin. Guava extracts have shown antimicrobial activity to a variety of pathogens associated with acute diarrhea (Iwu, 1995). Lutterodt (1989) demonstrated that alcoholic Soxhlet extracts of guava leaf inhibited both the spontaneous and electrically coaxially stimulated contraction of isolated guinea pig ileum. These results suggested that the anti-diarrheal activity of the extract is in part due to an inhibition of peristalsis. The inhibition is similar to that observed with morphine, one of the most effective clinically used drugs for the treatment of acute diarrhea. These results support the justification for the use of this plant in traditional medicine for the treatment of diarrhea.

The results of Table 9 and Table 10 demonstrate that the leaf extract of *S. incanum* inhibits the growth of all the stock cultures and eleven of the clinical isolates that it was tested against. Since the leaf extract has this antibacterial action against *E. coli*, *S. aureus*, *S. sonnei*, *S. dysenterica*, *V. cholera*, *S. typhimurium* and *S. typhi*, which are well-known toxin-producing bacteria associated with diarrheal diseases and dysentery one can easily justify its use in traditional medicine as a remedy for diarrhea, toothache, syphilis and abdominal pains, conditions which in one way or another are associated with bacterial infections. Results in Table 11 show that the plant extract contains volatile oils that are Well known for their demulcent and emollient properties, hence the use of this plant as a remedy for diarrhea and abdominal pains.

T minuta is a plant commonly used as a haemostatic and for treating wound infections. Its wound-healing property may lie in the fact that it has volatile oils, which are known to hinder bacterial growth and proliferation. The results summarized in Table 9 and Table 10 also show that *T minuta* has inhibitory effects on all the bacterial stock cultures and all the clinical isolates that it was tested against. It also has inhibitory effects on such bacteria as *E. coli*, *E. aerogenes*, *P. aeruginosa*, *S. aureus* and *P. vulgaris*, which are known to cause wounds This justifies the use of this plant as a wound healing agent in traditional medicine.

The results summarized in Tables 9 and 10 show that the leaf extract of *T. brachyceras* K. Schum. inhibited the growth of all the stock cultures and all the clinical isolates that it was tested against. The extract inhibited the growth of *S. aureus, E. coli, E. aerogenes* and *P. vulgaris* which comprise the bulk of microbial flora in the intestines and might cause constipation and other indigestion problems. This could justify the use of this plant as a remedy for constipation and other indigestion problems. The results summarized in Table 11 show that the plant contains anthracene glycosides which are well known for their laxative or purgative properties (depending on the dosage).

With a powerful effect, they act by stimulating peristaltic movements in the large intestines and thus diminishing water absorption. As a result, the transit of the faeces is quicker as they are less dry. Hence the use of this plant in the treatment of indigestion problems. The plant also contains volatile oils, which have a soothing effect on the skin. Herein lies the reason why the plant is used in the treatment of minor pains and itching in newborns.

Results summarized in Table 9 and Table 10 show that the leaf extracts of *V. auriculifera* (Welw.) Hiern. are inhibitory to the growth of all the stock cultures and the clinical isolates that they were tested against. *E. coli, E. aerogenes, P. aerogenes, S. aureus* and *P. vulgaris*, all of which are known to cause wounds are also inhibited. The results summarized in Table 11 show that *V. auriculifera* contains volatile oils, which are known to hinder the growth and proliferation of bacterial cultures. The results also show that the plant contains tannins, which are well known for their astringent properties. This is enough justification for the use of this plant in wound healing.

The results in Table 9 and Table 10 show that the leaf extracts of *H. fuscus* Garcke inhibited the growth of all the stock cultures and twelve of the clinical isolates that they were tested against. This could justify its use in the treatment of bacterial diseases. Results in Table 11 show that saponins, which are well known for their expectorant properties, are one of the phytoconstituents of this plant. Herein lies the justification for the use of this plant in the treatment of flu and cough.

Results in Table 9 and Table I0 indicate that the leaf extracts of *I. arrecta* A Rich have inhibitory effects against six of the bacterial stock cultures and four of the clinical isolates all of which are pathogenic, that they were tested against. This could explain the use of this plant as a remedy for stomachache. They had no action on *C. albicans* and nine of the clinical isolates. The results of Table 11 show that some of the phytoconstituents of *I. arrecta* include volatile oils, which have demulcent and emollient properties and are also known to hinder bacteria growth. Herein lies the justification for the use of this plant in traditional medicine as a remedy for stomachache.

Results in Table 9 and Table 10 show that the leaf/stem extract of *A. aspera* L. was inhibitory to all the bacterial stock cultures and all the clinical isolates that it was tested against but they had no action on *C. albicans*. The inhibition of all of which are known to cause wounds also inhibited helps to justify the use of this plant extract as a remedy for toothache, boils and abscesses. Results in Table 11 reveal that the plant contains fatty acids some of which can act as mild or strong purgatives and cathartics depending on the dosage. This justifies the use of this as a remedy for stomach problems. The results in Table 11 show that the plant contains saponins, which are well known for their expectorant properties. Their presence in this plant justifies its use as an emetic in traditional medicine and as a remedy for coughs.

The results in Table 9 and Table 10 reveal that leaf extracts of *A. conyzroides* L inhibited the growth of all the stock cultures and eleven of the clinical isolates that they were tested against. The results also reveal that *E. coli, P. aeruginosa, E. aerogenes, S. aureus* and *P. vulgaris*, all of which are known to cause wounds were also inhibited. The results in Table 11 show that *A. conyzoides* contains volatile oils, which are well known for their property of hindering bacterial growth and therefore, are generally useful in the treatment of wound infections. Volatile oils can also act as stomachics and are known to regulate intestinal movements by preventing or controlling violent contractions and aiding the orderly flow of food through the bowels. They are also useful as demulcents and emollients. Its use as eyewash for eyes can be deduced from its antibacterial activity and the presence of volatile oils.

Looking at the results of Table 9 and Table 10 it can be discerned that the leaf extract of *B. grantii* (Oliv.) Sheriff. inhibited the growth of all the stock bacterial cultures and twelve of the clinical isolates that it was tested against but they had no action on *C. albicans*. The antibacterial activity of this plant extract may explain its use as a remedy for stomach problems and pneumonia. A look at Table 11 shows that the plant contains volatile oils, which are well known for their property of hindering bacterial growth, regulation of peristaltic movements, demulcency and emolliency. This would be a good justification for its use in the treatment of stomach problems. The presence of saponins with their expectorant properties would justify their use as a cough remedy.

The Abagusii traditional healers are known to use *B. pilosa* in wound healing and as a styptic. The results summarized in Table 9 and Table 10 show very clearly that the leaf extracts of *B. pilosa* L. inhibited the growth of all the stock cultures and clinical isolates that they were tested against. The leaf extract also shows inhibitory effects on *E. coli, P. aeruginosa, E. aerogenes, S. aureus* and *P. vulgaris*. These coliform bacilli and Proteus are pathogens that are well known for causing approximately 40% of all nosocomial or hospital-acquired infections. The results in Table 11 reveal that *B. pilosa* contains volatile oils. These oils are known to hinder bacterial growth and they also act as emollients. Since the leaf extract of *B. pilosa* L. has shown antibacterial activity and has volatile oils, its use in wound healing is justified.

The results of Table 9 and Table 10 show that the leaf extracts of *S. didymobotrya* (Fresen) Irwin and Barnaby inhibited the growth of all the stock cultures and all the clinical isolates that were tested against it. This antimicrobial action alone would justify the use of this plant in the treatment of gonorrhea and stomach troubles. Looking at Table 9 it can be seen that the leaf extract of this plant inhibited the growth of *C. albicans*, a well-known fungal pathogen. This would explain the use of this plant in the treatment of ringworm fungal infections. Results of Table 11 show that the plant contains emodin, which is well known for its purgative action because of the anthraquinone molecule in its nucleus. This accounts for the purgative activity of this plant. The plant also contains volatile oils, which are well known for their antimicrobial action and the regulation of peristaltic movements. This may explain the use of this plant in the treatment of stomach problems.

The results in Table 9 and Table 10 that the leaf extracts of *C. vitellinum* (Benth) S. Moore inhibited the growth of all the stock cultures and the clinical isolates tested against it. This antimicrobial action would help explain the use of this plant in the treatment of a diseased eye (sore eye). The results in Table 11 show that the leaf extract of this plant gave a positive test for tannins which are Well known for their astringent properties and hence the use of this plant as a haemostatic.

The results of Table 9 and Table 10 show that the leaf extract of *D. integrifolia* (L.f.) O. Kuntze and an inhibitory effect on the growth of all the stock cultures and the clinical isolates tested against it. In addition, the inhibitory effect on the growth of *E. coli, P. aeruginosa, S. aureus, P. vulgaris,* which are all well-known as the causes of wounds could justify the use of this plant in traditional medicine as a wound healing agent. The results in Table 11 show that the leaf extract of this plant contains steroids/triterperroids and tannins. Tannins are well known for their astringent properties and isoprenoids such as steroids/ triterpenoids are known to contain volatile oils, which are Well known for their demulcent and emollient properties and the inhibition of bacterial growth. Hence the use of this plant in the treatment of thrush.

The results summarized in Table 9 and Table 10 show that an extract of the whole plant of *E. hirta* L. had inhibitory effects against all the stock cultures and the clinical isolates that they were tested against. *V. cholerae, E. coli, S. flaxineri, S. boydii, S. sonnei, S. dysenterica* and *S. aureus,* all bacterial species known to produce toxins associated with diarrheal diseases and dysentery were also inhibited. Herein lies the justification for the use of this plant in the treatment of diarrhea and dysentery. It also inhibits the growth of *E. aerogenes, S. aureus* and *P. vulgaris*, all Wound causing bacteria; hence the justification for its use as a remedy for thrush. Results in Table 11 reveal that the plant has the following phytoconstituents: steroids/ triterpenoids known to contain volatile oils, which are well known for the regulation of intestinal movements, preventing or controlling violent contractions and aiding the orderly flow of food through the bowel and inhibiting bacterial growth; tannins which are well known for their astringent action are also present. This is a confirmation of the antibacterial results that this plant is a useful remedy for diarrhea and dysentery.

A look at Table 9 and Table 10 shows the inhibitory effects of the root extract of *S tenuicarpa* Vollesen on all the stock cultures and ten of the clinical isolates that it was tested against. *E. coli, E. aerogenes, P. aeruginosa, S. aureus* and *P. vulgaris* bacterial species all well known for producing toxins that cause wounds were inhibited. Results in Table 11 show that an extract of this plant contains tannins, which are known for their astringent properties. This justifies the use of this plant as a wound-healing agent.

The results summarized in Table 9 and Table 10 show that the leaf extract of *R vulgaris* Meikle inhibited the growth of all the bacterial stock cultures and twelve of the clinical isolates that it was tested against but it had no action on *C. albicans*. *E. coli, E. aerogenes, P. aeruginosa, S. aureus* and *P. vulgaris*, all of which are known to be bacteria that cause wounds were among the inhibited species. Herein, lies the reason why this plant is a useful remedy in wound healing. Results from Tables 9 and 10 also show that the leaf extracts of this plant are inhibitory to the growth of *E. coli, E. aerogenes, S. aureus, P. vulgaris* and *S. tyuphimurium*. This antibacterial action of the leaf extracts would justify its use as a toothbrush. Because the extract is antibacterial to the above bacteria it will most likely be antibacterial in its action on the mouth micro-flora.

The results from the ethnomedical survey show that *R. vulgaris* has small edible fruits. It is well known that fruits are rich in vitamin C which is a preventive measure against scurvy. Hence the usefulness of this plant as a remedy for scurvy. Table 11 has results that show that the leaf extract of *R. vulgaris* contains tannins, which are well known for their astringent properties, hence the justification for the use of this plant in traditional medicine as a wound healing agent. The same leaf extract also contains volatile oils, which are known for their property of regulating intestinal movements, preventing or controlling violent contractions, aiding the orderly flow of food through the bowels and finally inhibiting the growth of bacteria. Herein lies the justification for the use of this plant in the treatment of diarrhea.

6.5 Medicinal and Poisonous Plants

Any medicine can be poisonous if taken in high doses. This means that the use of these medicinal plants should be done with caution. The Abagusii traditional medical practitioners know that plants such as *Gloriosa superba* L. (Liliaceae), *Cannabis saliva* L. (Cannabiaceae) and *Oxalis corniculata* L. (Oxalidaceae) have contraindications when used. They, therefore, advise on the judicious use of such plants by their patients. Medicinal plants contain various classes of compounds that include medicinal ones such as alkaloids and tannins. Some of these compounds are known to have bad side effects on human beings.

Alkaloids, for instance, have been implicated in both human and livestock poisonings. Over 6,000 plant species contain pyrrolizidine alkaloids (PA). This group of alkaloids constitutes one of the most important classes of toxicants of plant origin and may enter the human food supply as contaminants of grains and other foodstuffs, transferred through the food chain via consumption of animal products such as meat, milk, eggs and honey, occur as contaminants of herbal medicines, and be the active constituents of herbs used in herbal medicines and other herbal products.

The major problems associated with PA are found in three plant families -Boraginaceae, Compositae and Leguminosae. *Senecio longilobus* (Asteraceae) is poisonous to livestock and is notable for human toxicities arising from its accidental inclusion in herbal medicines The major toxic actions attributed to PA in humans are hepatic reno-occlusive disease, pulmonary arterial hypertension and right heart congestive failure (corpulmonale) and carcinogenesis. Many of the PAs are carcinogenic and this is of particular concern with the herb *Symphytum officinale* (Boraginaceae) which is widely consumed as a folk medicine.

The major plant genera associated with PA poisoning in humans are *Crotolaria* (Legurninosae), *Symphytum, Heliotropium* (Boraginaceae) and *Senecio* (Asteraceae). Poisoning from Crotalafia has been associated with the drinking of bush teas and contamination of grain crops in many countries

Comfrey (*Symphytum officinale*) is a herb to which almost supernatural powers are sometimes attributed. It has been credited with the ability to cause bone healing, cure cancer, "purify blood" and so on. Concern about the widespread consumption of comfrey tea and herbal products stems from the fact that comfrey contains several PAs.

A variety of other PA-containing plants could be items of the human diet. Borage (Borago officinalis) is a herb used in the preparation of salads or teas; it contains low levels of several PA, including lycopsamine which is hepatoxic and carcinogenic. The major problems of PA toxicosis in humans are attributable to poor fanning practices leading to the contamination of grain with toxic weed seeds and the use of herbal products.

Anthraquinone glycosides from various plants, especially from Cassia, *Rhamnus* and *Rheum* spp., are used as purgative preparations in traditional medicines. Anthraquinones are also employed as colourants, for instance in foods and drugs. The distribution of anthraquinones in edible and medicinal plants is less extensive than that of flavonoids, but it cannot be wholly discounted. The plants of the Polygonaceae, usually herbs, *Polygonium, Rheum, Rumex* etc., for example, *Rheum offinale* Baillon, *Rheum palmatum* L. or other species contain anthraquinone principles and emodin (a polyketide) and are used in traditional medicine as purgatives with secondary astringent action in indigestion; stomachic bitter and laxatives (Youngken, 1948). Traditional healers do not recommend excessive use of such plants, especially by young children. An extract from madder root (*Rubia tinctorum* L.) which has been used for the casing of ham and sausages in Japan, contains lucidin. This compound exhibited mutagenic and DNA-damaging properties (Yasui & Takeda, 1983).

Tannins are carcinogenic. Bracken fern has been found to contain carcinogenic tannins, which are, however, not the principal carcinogens of this plant. In addition, they are not carcinogenic when given orally. It was suggested that the consumption of tannin-rich herbal teas and medicines is responsible for the high incidence of esophageal cancer in many parts of the World (Morton, 1986). Coffee, cocoa and common tea are of particular significance to the total tannin load of humans. Among the beverages, common tea (*Cammellia sinensis* O. Kuntze) has the highest tannin yield. One cup of black tea may contain up to 500 mg. of tannins, depending on its origin and the mode of preparation. The tannin fraction of common tea was found to exhibit carcinogenic activity in rodents by subcutaneous injection. Although the carcinogenicity of tannins in animals and man is recommended for further study, they must be considered as potential carcinogens (Hiron, 1981; Lai & Woo, 1987; Concon, 1988; Pamukcu et al., 1980).

The importance of flavonoids as potential carcinogens stems from their widespread occurrence in human foodstuffs. Quercitin is one of the most common phenolic compounds in vascular plants. It occurs in fruits, vegetables and tea. Quercitin and several familiar flavonoids have been reported to be mutagenic in many short-term microbial assays (Brown, 1980).

Emodin (a polyketide) is mainly used as a cathartic. Although coumarin is a minor constituent of certain edible fruits (strawberries, cherries, apricots) and is present in many favouring agents, such as Lavendula (*Lavendula officinalis* Chaix), it has been reported that bile duct adenoma and carcinoma are induced in rats when fed diets containing 5000 ppm coumarin for prolonged periods. However, the experimental evidence for the carcinogenic activity of coumarin is rather limited (Lai & Woo, 1987; Concon, 1988).

The essential oils or terpenes from oranges, lemons, limes and grapefruit are carcinogenic, cocarcinogenic or tumour-promoting (Lei & Woo, 1987; Concon, 1988). The terpene fraction from orange oil, containing mostly D-limonene, gives rise to epidemic hyperplasia and eventually tumours (Lai & Woo, 1987; Condon, 1988).

Cyclopropane fatty acids are found in some plants of the order Malvales, for instance, cotton. Cotton seed oil from *Gossypium hirsutum* L. contains gossypol, a toxic and carcinogenic polyphenolic compound (Lai & Woo, 1987; Wogan & Busby, 1980; Concon, 1988; Ames, 1983).

Human populations throughout the world use many Euphorbiaceous plant species. Many of these plants have been reported to contain toxic phorbol esters, illustrating a potential environmental toxic hazard faced by people who come into direct contact with these species, either during the manufacture of products derived from these plants or direct exposure to the raw materials.

Some waxes and oils derived from the species of the neem tree are used in the manufacture of a variety of everyday products including soaps, cosmetics and medicines in Kenya. No toxicological/chemical investigations have been done on these chemicals. Currently, no governmental legislation exists for the control of the production of toxicological agents in commercially available products manufactured from this plant or any other plant. Therefore, attention needs to be given to the source of the production of these oils for inclusion in manufactured products if toxic effects are to be avoided.

The Cassava plant, *Manihot esculenta*; is used both as a medicinal and food plant although it has cyanogenetic glucosides that are poisonous and are known to give rise to several diseases (Poulton, 1983).

All species of the Cruciferae family that have been investigated contain one or more glucosinolates which are the precursors of compounds with goitrogenic action in mammals including humans (Bell & Belzile, 1965). The fleshy portion of some domesticated rosaceous species such as the apples, apricots and pears are non-cyanogenic; in contrast, the seeds enclosed may be highly cyanogenetic. Ingestion of such seeds has resulted in poisoning (Poulton, 1983).

It can be said that most medicinal herbs are not toxic as such and may be taken with less risk than any chemically synthesized medicine. To have medicinal effects, these plants must be administered in correct doses and correctly prescribed for the disease of the person taking them. It should be remembered that the same dose that heals an ill person might kill a healthy one.

During this study, it was revealed that traditional healers recommend the abstinence of certain foods by the patients. For example, the healers did not recommend the excessive use of certain plants during illness. This is in agreement with results found by other researchers (Bell & Belzile, 1965). It was found that traditional healers did not recommend excessive medication with plants such as tea. Although the traditional healers might not be aware of the scientific reasons behind their actions, their restriction of the excessive use of tannon-rich plants or any type of medicinal plants is justifiable.

Herbal products and folk medicines have had a mystique with the implication that since they are natural products, they must be good. Convincing the public that these products can be hazardous can be problematic.

However, the following guidelines are recommended for the effective use of herbs—they should never be given to babies a large quantity of any one of the preparations should not be taken and preparations which do not include a list of the plant constituents used should not be purchased.

Chapter Seven

Conclusions and Recommendations

7.1 Conclusions

The study demonstrated that the flora of Gusii land offers a largely untapped source of potentially useful medicinal plants. Numerous species are yet to be documented and investigated. The region also contains fungi, which could serve as excellent sources of bioactive substances. It is therefore important that measures are taken to conserve these fungi and other medicinal plants that in some cases are under threat of extinction. Cultures of these fruiting bodies of the fungi should be made and preserved. These fungal gene pools would enable the researchers to make available important strains on demand.

The results of this investigation have also supported the hypothesis that the plants used by Abagusii traditional medical practitioners have curative value. These results have revealed that there is a diversity of plants used by Abagusii healers. The results also show that the plants investigated have antimicrobial properties and chemical constituents that indicate their medicinal value. From these results, it was revealed that certain plants need to be used with caution because of their toxic properties. There is also a need to investigate the sustainability of the current practice of gathering plants in the wild. Because it was revealed in the study that medicinal plants are collected in different seasons there is a need to investigate the seasonability of the active principles. This seasonability may apply to some compounds but not to others. Herbal medicine should be seen as an important service to the people but more work is required to investigate the scientific basis of the practice.

In terms of in vitro inhibition of micro-organisms, this study was aimed at specific human pathogens. The approach differed from previous similar studies that aimed only at representative micro-organisms like gram-positive and gram-negative rods or cocci. All the plant extracts that were examined were found to contain different classes of active principles such as alkaloids, coumarins, tannins etc., that are known to be of medicinal value (Trease & Evans, 1978).

An important objective of this study and a significant aspect of the WHO's observation was the destruction of forests and the extinction of plant genetic pools. This is exemplified by the fact that new compounds that are effective in complicated disease conditions could be found in plants (Sheehan et al., 1992). It would also be good that in the search for bioactive compounds bioguided serendipity would be preferable over straight serendipity, i.e. exhaustive analysis of a plant sample for all types of natural products. It is evident that natural products have been and continue to be an important source of biologically active substances.

Finally, it is important to note that traditional medical practices should not be done away with but rather be improved on. Developing and applying scientific methodology to evaluate the medicinal value and document the physiological, pharmacological and toxicological properties of traditional drugs can do this. For the above to be achieved, there should be a working relationship between ethnobotanists, chemists, medical doctors, pharmacologists, pharmacists and traditional medical practitioners. This is because these are vital components of the stakeholders (research team).

Bearing in mind the great upsurge of interest in traditional plant medicines and the need to provide basic essential health care to every individual, one can confidently say that perhaps the greatest gain to be made in integrating traditional and orthodox systems of medicine into the official health care system of a developing nation is that the increase in manpower would help to provide total health coverage for all (WHO, 1978). This is because, after integration, some training for traditional medical practitioners (as well as legal control of their practice) must follow. Primary health care, at least would then be available to the whole population. It is at this level (and middle-level manpower) that the experiences of the traditional practitioner will be most useful.

The African Union (2001) and the WHO African Region (2001) have developed guidelines and protocols relating to policy, legal frameworks and research and development (R & D) methodologies on the promotion of traditional medicine and medicinal plants research in Africa for member states to adopt for use in their national strategic plans and programmes.

It is, therefore, recommended that toxicological studies of these plant extracts using suitable animal models be carried out to investigate their long-term effects. Otherwise from this investigation, it is proven that they kill micro-organisms and can be used against infections.

7.2 Recommendations

For research on traditional medicine and medicinal plants to continue conservation measures would have to be taken. These would include

7.2.1 Protection

Such measures as the proper harvesting of medicinal plants to avoid serious damage, the control of overgrazing and deforestation, protection of the sources of indigenous medicines such as forests, and salty rivers, allowing certain plants to rejuvenate, rotational grazing and the checking of bush encroachment by undesirable plant species.

7.2.2 Planting

Encouragement of small-scale cultivation of medicinal plants, thus leading to the conservation of gene pools, maintenance of mini forests on individual farms to increase biodiversity, the planting of medicinal plants on protected areas such as graveyards, church yards, institutions of higher learning and reserves, the incorporation of medicinal plants in agroforestry and reforestation programs, the encouragement of community actions to collect, retrieve and plant seeds of medicinal plants and the planting of medicinal plants on a commercial scale would be steps in the right direction.

The development of herbal or botanical gardens should also be encouraged. These gardens would provide a ready source of fresh material for ethnobotanical and phytopharmaceutical Work. If this is done, then it is possible to take the traditional doctors to the garden for the identification of the plants they use in the preparation of their phytomedicines. This will encourage traditional doctors and others to appreciate the medicinal significance of plant conservation

7.2.3 Legislation

Another conservation measure to be taken would be to legislate against the removal and export of rare species of medicinal plants i.e. strict control on the export of medicinal plants for commercial exploitation and the protection of the intellectual property rights (IPR) of traditional healers to encourage their practice

7.2.4 Research and Education

Research and education are important aspects of the conservation strategy of medicinal plants. The validation of the efficacy of traditional plants to gain user confidence is highly recommended. The promotion of public education on medicinal plants as the sources of modern medicine, the encouragement of the use of traditional plants and medicine in school curricula and higher institutions of learning and the development of new pharmacological methods and/or techniques for the screening of complex mixtures of plants such as decoctions, concoctions, crude drugs and extractives, since the fashionable methods of screening synthetic compounds are inadequate for a satisfactory evaluation of traditional medicines, are highly recommended.

Research in traditional medicine and medicinal plants. if aimed at the development of new drugs based on phytochemicals. must be interdisciplinary. It will involve a heterogeneous group of technical experts such as ethnobotanists, chemists, medical doctors, pharmacists, pharmacologists, toxicologists and traditional healers united in the application of their talents focused on a common object leading to the ensuring of a well-balanced research project on traditional medicine.

Such a research project should involve the socio-cultural aspects of traditional medicine. If such an approach were taken, it could reveal some information, which would lead to more understanding of traditional plant medicines that may result in unlimited potentialities and uninvestigated biodynamic activity from ethnomedical observations.

The preparation of a compendium of traditional treatment methods and methods for the standardization of herbal potions will need to be developed. This will eventually lead to the inclusion of medicinal plants/traditional medical recipes in official pharmacopoeias.

Attention must also be drawn to the fact that collaborative research will be necessary. Local industrial entrepreneurs will have to be involved in the above developments. This can be done through the attachment of their workers to traditional medicine research institutions. Eventually, this will attract them to start the manufacture of phytopharmaceuticals based on traditional medicines on modern lines. After all the above have been undertaken then traditional medicines are bound to replace to a large extent the expensive Western medicines thus making medical care, at least primary health care, to be within the reach of one and all by the year 2010 (AU, 2001).

References

Addae- Mensah. I, Torto, F. G., Dimonyelca, C. 1., Baxter, I. & Sanders, J. K.M.(1977). Novel amide alkaloids from the roots of *Piper guineense. Phytochemistry* **16**: 757.

Adesanya, S.A and Roberts, M.F. (1995). Inducible compounds in *Phaseolus, Vigna* and *Dioscorea* species in *Handbook of phytoalexin metabolism and action* (eds, M. Daniel and R. Purkayastha): 333-373. Marcel Dekker, New York.

African Union (2001). *Decade for African Traditional Medicine* (2001-2010) (*AU/AHG Dec. 164 XXXVII, 2001*) Lusaka: 171-174.

Akpata, L. (1979). The practice of herbalism in Nigeria. In: *African Medicinal Plants* (ed. Sofowora, E. A.) University of Ife Press, Ife, Nigeria: 13-20.

Akunyili, D.N., Houghton, P. J. & Raman, A. (1991). Antimicrobial activities of the stem bark of *Kigelia pinnata. Journal of Ethnopharmacology* **35**: 173-177.

Alade, P. I. & Irobi, O. N. (1993). Antimicrobial activities of crude leaf extracts *of Acalypha wilkesiana. Journal of Ethnopharmacology* 39: 1-9.

Ames, B.N. (1983). Dietary carcinogens and anticarcinogens. *Science* **221**: 1256.

Amponsah-Agyemang, G. (1980). The use of plants in traditional medical practice in an Ashante village. B.Sc. Thesis. Institute of Renewable Natural Resources, University of Science and Technology, Kumasi, Ghana.

Anyigwo, C.E. (1986) The anti-bacterial effect of the essential oil of *Ocimum gratissimum. Journal of Research on Ethnomedicine* **1(1)**: 4-8.

Balandalin, M.F., Klocke, J.A., Wurtele, E.S. & Bollinger, W.H. (1985). Natural plant chemicals: sources of industrial and medicinal materials. *Science* **228**: 1154-1160.

Barrett, J. A (1996): *The Turkana and their trees; Their medical and ecological value.* Kenya Litho, Kenya.

Bauer, A. W., Kirby, W. M., Shervis, J.C. & Turk, M. (1996). Current techniques for antibiotic susceptibility. *American Journal of Clinical Pathology* **45**: 493.

Bell, J.M & Belzile, R. J. (1965) *Goitrogenic properties in rapeseed meal for livestock and poultry: a review* (eds Bowlzmd, J. P., Clandinin, D. R, & Wetter, L. R.) Canada Department of Agriculture

Braquet, P., & Hysoford, D. (1991). Ethno pharmacology and the development of natural PAF antagonists as therapeutic agents. *Journal of Ethno pharmacology* **32**:135-149.

Brenan, J. P. M. (1949). *Check list of trees and shrubs of Tanganyika Territory.* Imperial Forestry Institute, Oxford.

Bringmann, G., Grarnatokis, S., & Proksch, P. (1992). Feeding deterrency and growth retarding activity of the thylisoquinoline alkaloid dioncyphylline A against *Spodoptera littoralis. Phytochemistry* **31: (3)**: 821-3 825.

Bringmann, G, Scheneider C. 1-1, Polcorny, F., Loren; H., & Fleischmann, H., (1996) African plants as sources of pharmacologically exciting biaryl and quartenaryl alkaloids. In: *Chemistry, biological and pharmacological properties of African medicinal plants*: (ed. Hostettman K.): 1-19.

Brown, J.P. (1980) A review of the genetic effects of naturally occurring flavonoids, anthraquinones and related compounds. *Mutagenic Research* **75**: 243.

Caceras, A. A, Fletes, L. Aguilar, L.& Ramirez, D. (1993). Plants used in Guatemala for the treatment of gastrointestinal disorders: Confirmation of activity against Enterobacteriaceae. *Journal of Ethnopharmacology* **38:(3)**: 1-3 8.

Chang, H. M. & But, P.P.H. (1987) *Pharmacology and applications of Chinese material medica Vols 1&2*, Singapore, World scientific Publications: 1-1320.

Chhabra, S.C., Shao, T.F., Mshiu, E.N & Uiso, F.C. (1981). Screening of Tanzanian medicinal plants for antimicrobial activity. *Journal of African Medicinal Plants* **4**: 93-98.

Chhabra, S. C., Uiso, F. C. & Mshiu, E. N. (1984). Phytochemical screening of Tanzanian Medicinal Plants. *Journal of Ethnopharmacology* **11**: 157-179.

Chhabra, S.C., Muregi, F. W., Njagi, E. N. M, Langat-Thoruwa, C. C., Njue, W.M, Orago, A. S. S., Omar, S. A. & Ndiege, I. O. (2003). *In vitro* antiplasmodial activity of some plants used in Kisii, Kenya against malaria and their chloroquine potentiation effects. *Journal of Ethnophannacology* **84**: 235-239.

Concon, J.M., (1988). *Food Toxicology*, Part A: Principles and Concepts. Marcel Dekker, New York, Chapter 8.

Dalziel, J. M., (1956). *The Useful Plants of West Tropical Africa*. Crown Agents, London.

Department of Forest Genetics and Plant Physiology, Swedish University of Agricultural Sciences.

Ellis, H.& Calne, RY. (1977). *Lecture Notes on General Surgery*, 5th ed. Blackwell Scientific Publications, Oxford.

El-Said, F., Sofowora, E. A., Malcolm, S. A. & Hofer, A. (1969). An investigation into the efficacy of *Ocimum gratissimum* (L.) as used in Nigerian native medicine. *Planta Medica*, **17**: 195.

Encarnacion, R. & Gaza, S.K. (1991) Antimicrobial screening of medicinal plants from Baja, California Sur, Mexico. *Journal of Ethnopharmacology* **31**: 181-192.

ENDA, 1987. Environment afiicain: série plantes médicinales. Fiche technique. ENDA (Environment ET Development du Tiers Moncle), Dakar, Senegal.

Fellows, L. E. (1992). Pharmaceuticals from traditional medicinal plants and others: future prospects. In: *New drugs from natural sources*. London, IBC Technical Services.

Francois, G., Bringmann, G., Phillipson, J.d., Ake' Assi, L., Dochez, C., Rubenacker, M., Scheneider, Ch., Wery, M, Warhnrst, D.C., & Kirby, G.C.(l994). Activity of extracts and naphthyliisoquinoline alkaloids from *Triphyophyllum peltatum, Ancistrocladus abbreviatus and A. barteri against Plasmodium falciparum* in in vitro. Phytochemistry **35**: 1461-1464.

Galloway, J.H., Marsh, I. D., & Bittiner, S.B. (1991) Chinese herbs for eczema: The active compound? *Lancet* **337**: 566.

Gbile, Z.O. & Adensia, S.K. (1987). Nigeria pharmaceutical potentials. *Journal of Ethnopharmacology* **19 (1)**: 1-17.

Gelfand, M., Mavi, S., Drummond, R. B., & Nclemera, B. (1985) *The Traditional Medical Practitioner in Zimbabwe.* Mambo Press, Harare.

Gessler, M. C., Nkunya, M. H. H., Mwasumbi, L. B., Heinriclg M., & Tanner, M. (1994) Screening Tanzanian Plants for antimalarial activity. *Acta Tropica* **56**: 65-6'7.

Grein, E. & Brantner, A. (1994) Antibacterial activity of plant extracts used externally in traditional medicine. *Journal of Ethnopharmacology* **44**: 35-40.

Gruenweller, S., Schroeder, E. & Juergen, K. (1990). Biological activities of furastanol saponins from Nicotiana tabacum. *Phytochemistry* (Oxl) **29(8)**: 2485-2490.

Gundidza, M & Gaza, N. (1993). Antimicrobial activity of *Dalbergia melanoxylon* extracts. *Journal of Ethnopharmacology* **40**: 127-130.

Hiron, I. (1981). Natural carcinogenic products of plant origin. *CRC Critical Review of Toxicology* **8**: 235.

Hostettmann, K., & Hostcttmann, M., (1989) Xanthones. In: *Methods of Plant Biochemistry* (eds. J. B. Harborage): 493-508. Academic Press, London.

Hostettmann, K., Marston, A. & Wolfender, J. L. (1995) Strategy in the search for new biologically active plant constituents. In: *Phytochemistry of Plants used in Traditional Medicine* (Eds. K. Hostettmann, K. Marston, M. Maillard & Hamburger, M), Oxford Science Publications Oxford: 17-45.

Hostettmann K. (1978), Inhibition of type A and type B monoamine oxidase by isogentisin and its 3-0- glucoside. *Biochemical Pharmacology* **27**: 2075-2078.

Hussein, N., Modan, M.H., Shabbir, S. G. & Zaidi, AH. (1979). Antimicrobial principles in *Mimosa humata. Journal of Natural Products* **42(5)**: 525-527.

Irobi, O.N. & Daramola, S.O. (1993). Antifungal activities of crude extracts of *Mitracarpus villosus* (Rubiaceae). *Journal of Ethnopharmacology* **40**: 137-140.

Irobi, O.N. & Daramola, S.O. (1994). Bactericidal properties of crude extracts of *Mitracarpus villosus* (Rubiaceae). *Journal of Ethnopharmacology* **42**: 39-43.

Ikan, R. (1969) Natural Products: A Laboratory Guide. Academic Press, London.

Iwu, M.M. (1995) *Handbook of African medicinal plants*. CRC Press, Bcca, Raton.

Jawetz, E., Melnick, IL. & Adelberg, E.A. (1970). *Review of Medical Microbiology*. San Francisco U.S.A.: 194.

Johansson, S. G., Alakoski-Johansson, G. M., Luukkanen, O.M., Mulatya, J& Gachathi, N (1987). Ethnobotanical approach to seed procurement: experience from Bura, Kenya. In: *Proceedings of the International Symposium on forest seed problems in Africa*. Report 7. (eds S.K. Kamra & R.D. Ayling)

Johansson, S. G., & Alalcoski~Iol1anssorL G. M. (1988) Ethnobotanical Research and rural development experiences from the Bum Forestry Research Project. *Silva carelica* **12**:263-269.

Johns, T., Kokwaro, J.O. & Kimanani, E.K. (1990). Herbal remedies of the Luo of Siaya District, Kenya; Establishing criteria for consensus. *Economic Botany* **44 (3)**:369-381.

Kerharo, J. & Adams, J. G. (1974) *La Pharmacopee Senegalese Traditionnelle*. Vigot, Paris.

Kinghorn, A. D. & Balandilin, M. F., (1993). *American Chemical Society Symposium Series*, 539: 1-348.

Kioy, D.W. (1989). A study of the chemistry and pharmacology of phytochemicals from three species of *Canellaceae*. Ph.D. thesis, University of Strathclyde, Scotland: 241.

Kleyn, J. & Hough, J. (1971). The microbiology of brewing. *Annual Review of Microbiology* **25**: 583.

Kokwaro, J. O. (1991). Conservation of medicinal plants. *Proceedings of an International Consultation 21st -27th March 1988*. Thailand: 315-319.

Kokwaro, J.O. (1993). *Medicinal plants of East Africa*. East African Literature Bureau Kampala, Nairobi, Dar-Es-salaam.

Kubo, I & Taniguchi, M. (1988). Polygodial antifungal potentiator. *Journal of Natural Products* **51**: 22-29.

Kubo, I., Himejima, M., Tsujimoto, K. & Muroi, H. (1992). Antibacterial activity of crinitol and its potentiation. *Journal of Natural Products* **55(6):** 780-785.

Lai, D.Y. & Woo, Y. (1987). Naturally occurring carcinogens: an overview: Environment carcinogenicity Review (*Journal of Environmental Science & Health*) **C5(2) 121**:121.

Lambo, J. O. (1979). The healing powers of herbs with special reference to obstetrics and gynaecology. In: *African Medicinal Plants* (ed. Sofowora, E. A.). University of Ife Press, lfe, Nigeria: 23-31.

Le Strange, R. (1977) *A History of Herbal Plants.* Angus & Robertson, London.

Lindsay, R. S. (1978). *Medicinal plants of Marakwet, Kenya.* Royal Botanic Gardens, Kew.

Luttge, U. & Smith, I. AC. (1982). Membrane transport, Osmoregulation and the Control of CAM. In: *Crassulacean Acid Metabolism* (eds. I. P. Ting & M. Gibbs): 69-91. American Society of Plant Physiology, Rockville.

Lutterodt, G.D. &Maleque, A. (1989). Effect on mice locomotor activity of a narcotic-like principle from guava leaves. *Journal of Ethnopharmacology* **24**: 219-231.

MacGregor, E. & Greenwood, C. (1980). *Polymers in Nature.* John Wiley & Sons, Chichester.

Magro-Filho, O. & de Carvallo, A. C. (1994). Topical effect of propolis in the repair of sulcoplasties by the modified Kayanjian technique: Cytological and Clinical evaluation: *Journal of Nihom University School of Dentistry* **36:** 102-111.

Makhubu, L. P. (1978) *The Traditional Healer.* The University of Botswana and Swaziland Press, Kwaluseni, Swaziland.

Marston, A. & Hostemann, K. (1987) Antifungal, molluscicidal and cytotoxic compounds from plants used in traditional medicine. In: *Biologically active natural products: Proceedings of the Phytochemical Society of Europe Vol. 27* (Eds. K. Hostettmann & P.J. Lea): 65-83. Oxford Science Publication. Oxford.

Maundu, P. M. Ngugi, G. W. & Kabuye, C. H. S (1999). Kenya Resource Centre for Indigenous Knowledge, National Museums of Kenya, Nairobi.

McCutcheon, A.R., Ellis, S. M., Hankock, R.E.W.& Towers, G_H.N. (1992). Antibiotic screening of medicinal plants of the British Colombian native peoples. *Journal of Ethnopharmacology* **37**(3): 213-223.

McDowell, P.G., Lwande, W., Deans, S.G. & Waterman, P.G. (1988). Volatile resin exudates from the stem bark of *Commiphora rostrata*: Potential role in plant defence. *Phytochemistry* **27(8)**: 2519-2521.

Mensah, I.A. and Achenbach, L.T. (1987): *Rationalizing traditional medicine: Some recent research with a symposium on appropriate technology in disease control: Proceedings of the 8th Annual Medical Scientific Conference,* Nairobi, Kenya: 151-154.

Mitscher, L.A., Showalter, H.D.H., Shipchandler, M.T., Len, R.P., Beal, J.L. (1972). Antimicrobial agents from higher plants. IV: *Zanthoxylum elephantiasis*: Isolation and identification of Canthin-6-one. *Lloydia* **35(2)**: 177-180.

Mitscher, L.A., Drake, S. Colladi S.R_ & Okwute, S.K. (1987). A modern look at folklore use of anti-infective agents. *Journal of Natural Products* **50**: 1025.

Mizuo, M., Iinuma, M., Tanaka, T., Iwashima, S., Sakaribara, N., Liu, X. S., Shi, D & Muessel, H. (1990) Flavonal glycosides and their distribution in the leaves of the genus *Epidium. Asian Journal of Plant Science* **1(1):** 1-6.

Morgan, W.T. W. (1980) *Vernacular names and the utilization of plants among the Turkana of Northern Kenya. Special Report,* Department of Geography, University of Durham.

Morgan, W.T. W. (1981) *Ethnobotany of the Turkana: use of plants by a pastoral people and their livestock in Kenya. Economic Botany* **35**: 96-130.

Morris, E. J., Dowler, S., & Cullen, B. (1994). Early clinical experience with topical collagen in vascular wound care. *Journal of Wound Ostomy and Continence Nursing* **21**; 247-250.

Morton, J. F. (1986). The potential carcinogenicity of herbal tea. *Environmental Carcinogenicity Review (Journal of Environmental Science & Health)* **C4 (2)**: 203.

Mott, K. E. (1987). *Plant Mollucicides.* Wiley, Chichester.

National Drug Policy (NDP, 1993). Ministry of Health. Government Printer. Nairobi.

Ogol, C. K. P. 0., Ogola, P. 0., Odede, W. D. & Khayota, B. (2002).

Indigenous knowledge of medicinal and plants of Mfangano Island, Lake Victoria, Kenya. *East African Journal of Science* **4(1)**; 11-28.

Ogunyemi, O. (1979) The origin and spread of herbalism in Nigeria. In: *African Medicinal Plants* (Ed. Sofowora, E. A) University of Ife Press, Ife, Nigeria: 10.

Ojewole, J.A & Adesina, S.K. (1983). Cardiovascular and neuromuscular achons of Scopoletin from the fruits of *Tetrapleura tetreptera*. *Planta Medica* **49**: 99-102.

Okemo, P.O. (1996). Antimicrobial efficacy of selected medicinal plants used by Kenyan herbal doctors. Ph.D. Thesis, Kenyatta University, Nairobi, Kenya: 173-190.

Okemo, P.O. & Mwatha, E. W. (2002). In vitro activity of selected medicinal plant extracts against pathogenic bacteria and HIV/ AIDS-related *Mycobacterium* spp. *Journal of Tropical Microbiology* **1**: 30-36

Oligashi, H., Takagaki, T., Koshimizzi, K, Watunabe, K., Kaji, M., Hoshino, J., Nashids, T. & Hufinan, M. A. (1991). Biological activities of plant extracts from Tropical Africa. *African Study Monographs* **12(4)** :201-210.

Oliver, B. (1959). *Medicinal Plants in Nigeria*. Nigerian College of Arts, Science and Technology.

Onawumni, G.O., Yisak, W., & Ogunlana, E.O. (1984). Antimicrobial constituents in the essential oil of *Cymbopogon citratus* (DC) Stapf. *Journal of Ethnopharmacology* **12**: 279-286.

Organization of African Unity (OAU) / Scientific and Technical Committee (STRC). Dakar (1968). *First Inter-African Symposium on Traditional Pharmacopoeia and African Medicinal Plants*. Publication No. 104. OAU/STRC, Lagos

Organization of African Unity(OAU)/Scientific and Technical Committee (STRC).

Second Inter-African Symposium on Traditional Pharmacopoeia and African Medicinal Plants. OAU Publication No. 115. OAU/STRC. Dakar (1979), Lagos: 43-49.

Padmaja, V., Thankmany. V. & Hisham, A. (1993). Antibacterial, antifungal and antihelmintic activities of root barks of *Uvaria lookeri and Uvaria narum. Journal of Ethnopharmacology* **40**: 181-186.

Pamukcu, A.M., Wang, C. Y., Haicher, J. 8: Bryan, G.T. (1980) Carcinogenicity of tannin and tannin free extracts of bracken fern (*Pteridium aquilinum*) in rats. *Journal of National Cancer Institute* **65**: 131.

Parr, A. J., Payne, J., Eagles, T., Chapman, B.T., Robbins, R J. & Rhodes, M. J. C. (1990) Variation in tropane alkaloid accumulation within the Solanaceae and strategies for its exploitation. *Phytochemistry* (Oxf) **29(8)**: 2545-2550.

Paulo, M.Q., Barbosa-Filho, J.M., Lima, E.O., Maia, R.F, & Cassia, R. (1992). Antimicrobial activity of benzylisoquinoline alkaloids from *Annona salzmanii* DC. *Journal of Ethnapharmacology* **36**: 39-41.

Penera, P.T., Vitkova, A & Ivancheva, S. (1988) Santonin, essential oils and flavonoid content in *Artemisia santonicum* L. Rasteniv' 'd Nauki **25(7)**: 35-42.

Phillipson, J.D., Wright, C. W., Kirby, G.C.& Warhurst, D. C., (1993): *Tropical plants as sources of antiprotozoal agents*. New York, Plenum: 1-40.

Pomilio, A. B., Buschi, C_A., Tomes, C.N. and Viale, A. A (1992). Antimicrobial constituent of *Gomphrena martiana* and *Gomphrena boliriana. Journal of Ethnopharmacolog* **36**; 155-161.

Poulton, J. E. (1983). Cyanogenic compounds in plants and their toxic effects in: *Handbook of Natural Toxins 1*: 117 (Eds: Keeler, R.F & Tu, T. A.). Marcel Dekker, New York.

Rodriguez, Si, Wolfender, J. L., Hakizamungu, E., & Hostettmann, K (1995). An antifungal napthoquinone, xanthones and seroiridoids from *Swertia calycina. Planta Medica* **61**:3362-3 64.

Rogers, C.B. (1989a). Isolation of the 1 & hydroxy cycloartenoid mollic acid and L-arabinoside from *Commbretum edwardii* leaves. *Phytochemistry.* **28**: 528-533.

Rogers, C.B. (1989b). New mono-and bi-desmosidic triterpenoids isolated from *Combretum padoides* leaves. *Journal of Natural Products.* **52**: 528-533.

Ross, M.S.F. & Brain, K.R (1977). *An Introduction to Phytopharmacy.* Pitman Medical, Kent.

Rowe, T.D.E, Lovell, B.K. & Parks, L.M. (1941). Further observations on the use of *Aloe vera* leaf in the treatment of third-degree X-ray reactions. *Journal of the American Pharmaceutical Association* **29**: 266-269. Scientific Edition.

Sahle, S & Gashe, B.A (1991). The microbiology of Tella fermentation. *SINET: Ethiopian Journal of Science* **14**: 93.

Sainsbury, M., & Sofowora, E. A. (1971) Essential oils from the leaves and inflorescence of *Ocimum gratissimum. Phytochemistry* 10(8): 3309.

Sakanaka, S., Kim, M., Taniguchi, M. & Yanamoto, T. (1989). Antimicrobial substances in Japanese green tea extract against *Streptococcus mutants,* a cariogenic bacterium. *Agricultural Biological Chemistry* **53(9):** 2307-2311.

Sakaranarayanan, A.S., Almeida, M.R. Govindachari, T.R. & Ake Assi, L. (1993). The cultivation of tropical lianas of genus *Ancistrocladus. Planta Medica* **(59) {Suppl. 1}**: 623-624.

Schafelberger, D. & Hostettmann, K. (1988) Chemistry and pharmacology of *Gentiana lacteal: Plant Medica* **54**: 219- 221.

Sheehan, M.P., Rustin, M.H.A. & Atherton, D.J. (1992). The efficiency of traditional Chinese herbal therapy in adult atopic dermatitis: Results of a double-blind placebo-controlled study. *Lancet* **34**: 13-17.

Shengj-ji, P.E. I. (1989). Preliminary S1lICll6S on the edible flowers of Northwest Yunan (China). Asian *Journal of Plant Science* **1(2)**: 69-78.

Sofowora, F. A (1982). *Medicinal plants and traditional medicine in Africa.* John Wiley and Sons, N.Y, U.S.A.

Sofowora, F.A. (1996). *Plantes medicinales et medicine traditionalle d'Afrique*, Karthala, Paris.

Solecki (1975). Shanida IV. A Neanderthal flower burial in Northern Iraq. *Science* **190**: 880-881,

Takeshi, K., Yamane, F. & Morita, Y. (1990) Flavanol glycosides and other constituents from the leaves of *Ampelopsis brevipedunculata* Trautv. *Shoyakugaku Zasshi* **44(2)**: 138-142.

Tanake J. (1983). List of plants collected from Baringo, Elgeyo Marakwet and West Pokot Districts. Appendix X: 147-164. In: Kerio Valley: past, present and future: *Proceedings of seminar, Institute of African Studies*, University of Nairobi.

Taniguchi, H. & Kubo, I. (1993) Ethno botanical drug discovery based on medicine men's trials in the African Savanna: Screening of East African plants for antimicrobial activity II: *Journal of Natural Products* **56(9)**: 1539-1546.

Tanira M.O.M., Bashir, A. Dib. R, Godwin C.S. Wasti, I. A & Banna, N. R. (1994). Antimicrobial and phytochemical screening of medicinal plants of the United Emirates. *Journal of Ethnopharmacology* **41**; 201-205.

Taylor, X. (1965). *Plant Drugs that Changed the World*. George Allen & Unwin Ltd.

TDR (Research and Training in Tropical Diseases) (2000) News.

Tessema, A. D. (1994). Ph. D. Dissertation, Moscow State Academy of Food Products, Moscow.

Thomson, A. R. W. (1980) (Ed). *Healing plants*. Macmillan, London Limited.

Timberlake, J. R. (1987) *Ethnobotany of the Pokot of Northern Kenya*. East African Herbarium, Nairobi.

Ting, I. P. (1985) Crassulacean Acid Metabolism. *Annual Review of Plant Physiology* 36: 5 95-622.

Trease, G. E & Evans, W. C (1987). *Pharmacognosy*. Bailliére- Tindall, London

White, N. J., Waller, D., Crawley, J., Nosten, F., Chapman, D.& Greenwood, B.M.(1992). Comparison of artemether and chloroquine for severe malaria in Gambian children, *Lancet* **339**:317-321.

UNIDO (1978). Technical Consultation on the production of drugs from medicinal plants in developing countries. *UNIDO Document NO. ID/ 22(ID/ WG 271?6)*.

USN (United States Navy, Navy Medical Department) (2001). *Guide to malaria prevention and control*. Navy Environmental Health Centre, Norfolk.

Watt, J. M. & Breyer-Brandwijk, M, G. (1962), The medicinal and poisonous plants of Southern and Eastern Africa. 2nd ed. E and S. Livingstone Ltd, Edinburgh; London.

Wogan G. N. & Busby, W. F. Jr. (1980) Naturally occurring carcinogens. In: *Toxic Constituents of Plant Foodstuffs*, 2nd edn., (Ed, Liener, I.E.), Academic Press, New York. Chapter 11.

World Health Organization (WHO) (1976). Resolution- Health Manpower Development. *WHO Document No. WHA.29.72.*

WHO (1977). Resolution- Promotion and Development of Training and Research in Traditional Medicine. *WHO Document No. WHA 30.49*

WHO. (1978) Resolution- Drug Policies and Management of Medicinal Plants. *WHO Document No. WHA 31.33*

WHO (1978 a). Health Manpower Development: Training and Utilization of Traditional Healers and their Collaboration with Health Care Systems. *WHO Document No. EB 57/21 Add 2.*

WHO. (1978). The promotion and development of Traditional Medicine, *Technical Report Series, No. 622,* Geneva.

WHO (1970). Resolution- Traditional Medicine Programme. *WHO Document No. EB 63. R 4.*

WHO. (1998) Roll back malaria. *Fact Sheet No. 203.* WHO, Geneva

WHO. (2000*) Severe Falciparum Malaria Transactions of the Royal Society of Tropical Medicine and Hygiene* **94 (Suppl. 1)**: 36-37.

WHO (2001). *Promoting the Role of Traditional Medicine in Health Systems; A Strategy for the African Region (AFR/RC 509).* Regional Office for Africa

Wrangham, R.W., (1975). The behavioural ecology of chimpanzees in Gombe National Park, Tanzania Ph.D. Thesis. The University of Cambridge.

Wrangham, R.W., & Goodhall (1989), I. Chimpanzee use of medicinal leaves in: *Understanding chimpanzees (eds:* P.G. Helne and L.A. Marquardt). Cambridge; Harvard University Press: 22-37

Wright, C. & Phillipson, J. D. (1990), Natural Products and Development of Selective Antiprotozoal Drugs. *Phytotherapy Research* **4**:127-139.

Yasui, Y. & Takeda, N. (1983) Identification of a mutagenic substance in *Rubia tinctorum* L. (madder) root as lucidin. *Mutagenic Research* **121**:185.

Youngken, H.W. (1948). *Textbook of Pharmacognosy.* McGraw-Hill Book Company, Inc., New York, Toronto, London

Zucker, J.R. & Campbell, C. C. (1993) Malaria: Principles of prevention and treatment *Infectious Disease Clinics of North America* **7**: 547-567.

APPENDIX - QUESTIONNAIRE

Information Required on Plants of Medicinal Value

(One form to be completed for each plant)

Researcher ....

Name and address of institution ....

Date ....

Traditional Medicine Plant Collection Number (TMP No.) ....
....

1. Family ....

2. Genus and species ....

3. Vernacular name(s). ....

4. Disease(s) for which the plant is a remedy (Be as specific as possible)

   ....
   ....
   ....
   ....

5. Plant part(s) used

   ....

6. Method(s) of preparation for use (Provide details about the amount of plant part(s) required), whether fresh or dried, ratio of plant to medium of preparation, etc. (For additional information use an extra paper)

   ....
   ....

....

....

7. Mode of administration (including dosage) ....
......

8. Other plants or ingredients with which the plant is used for the preparation: State genus, species, and family, the vernacular name and the part used

....

....

....

....

9. Can the preparation be made in any other way, e.g. using another medium e.g. *busaa*, local gin, etc. instead of water? *Yes/No. If yes, give details*

....

....

....

....

....

10. Name and address of the Traditional Medical Practitioner or any other person giving the information about the medicinal value of the plant.

....

....

....

....

11.Any other remarks e.g. time of collection, where to collect, etc.

....

....

....

....

Plant Images

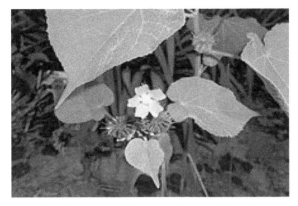

Abutilon mauritiunum (Omorobianda)

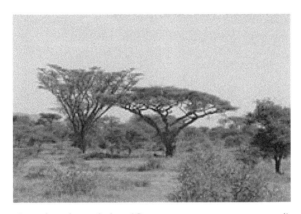

Acacia abyssinica (Omonyenya omwegarori)

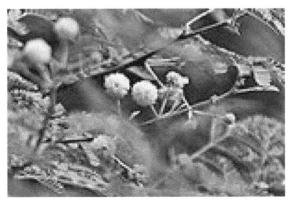

Acacia nilotia (Omonyenya)

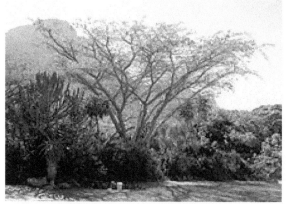

Acacia sieberiana (Eyesura)

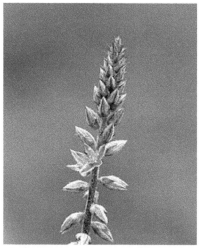

Achyranthes aspera (Esarara)

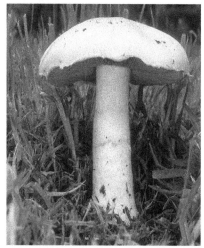

Agaricus campestris (Oboba)

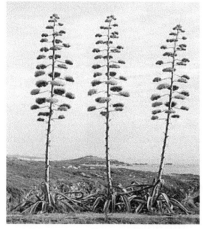

Agave americana (Rikonge)

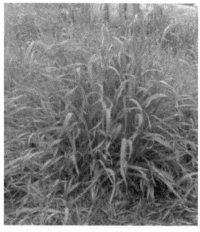

Agropyron repens (Ekenyambi)

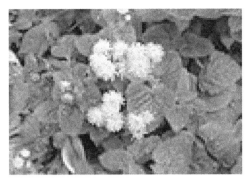

Ageratum conzyoides (Emete y'amaiso)

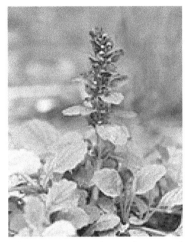

Ajuga remota (Omosinyonta)

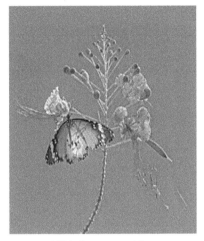

Albizia gummifera
(Omogonchoro)

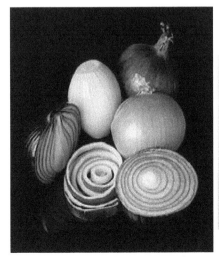

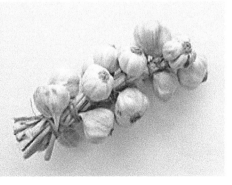

Allium sativum (Egetunguo saumu)

Allium cepa (Egetunguo)

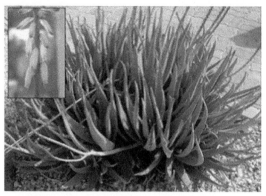

Aloe vera (L.) Burm (Omogaka)

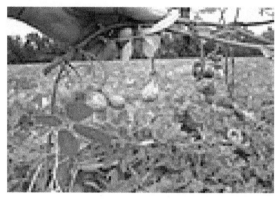

Arachis hypogea (Chinchugu)

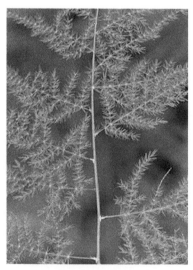

Asparagus africanus
(Ekerobo)

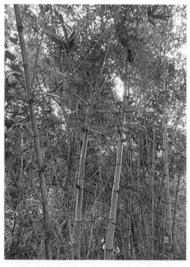

Bambusa vulgaris (Emoti)

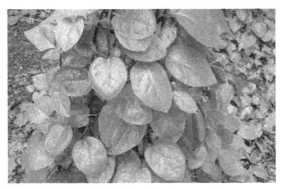

Basella alba (Enderema)

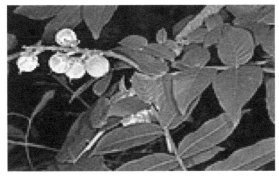

Bersema abyssinica (Omobamba)

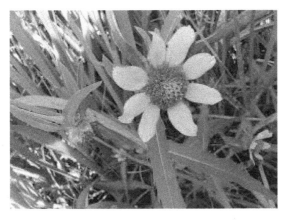

Bidens grantii (Rirarang'era)

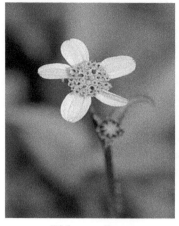

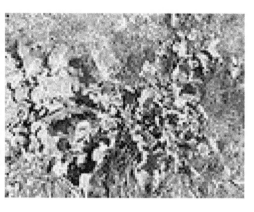

Bidens pilosa
(Ekemogamogia)

Brassica oleraceae (Ekabichi
nyamato)

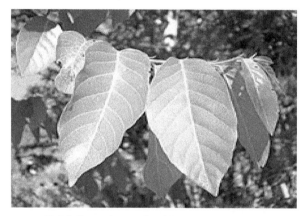

Bridelia micrantha (Omotaraganga)

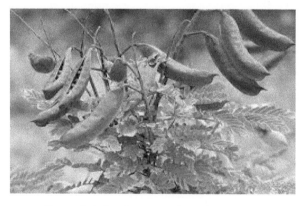

Caesalpinia decapetala (Ekenagwa)

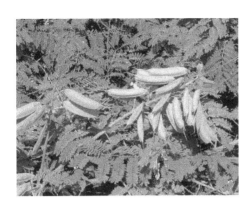

Caesalpinia decapetala (Ekenagwa)

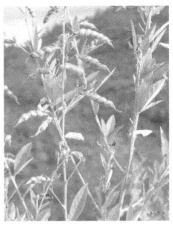

Cajuns cajan (L.) Millsp.
(Chimbisi)

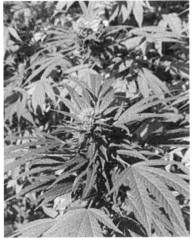

Cannabis sativa (Enyasore)

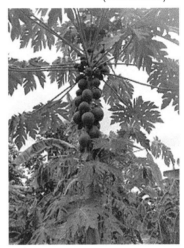

Carica papaya (Ripaipai)

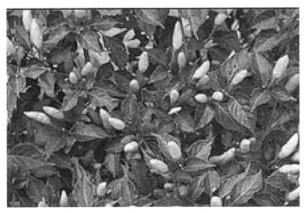

Capsicum frutescens (Earare)

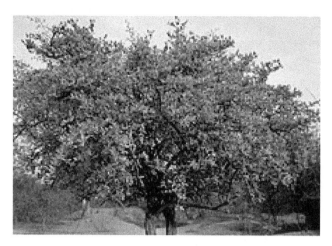

Carissa edulis (Omonyangateti)

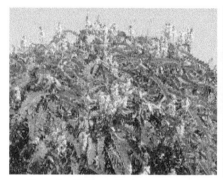

Cassia didymobotyra Fresen
(Omobeno)

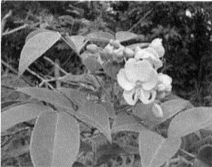

Cassia floribunda (Omobeno
omwegarori)

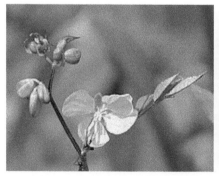

Cassia occidentalis (Omote
ogotioka)

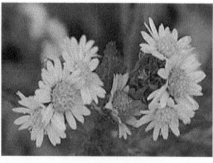

Chrysanthemum cineriaefolium
(Riuga)

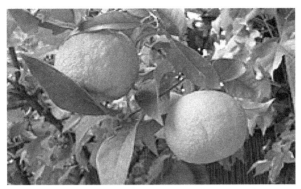

Citrus aurantium (Ritunda riroro)

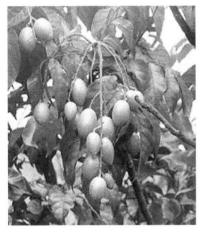

Clausena anisata
(Omonyansuri)

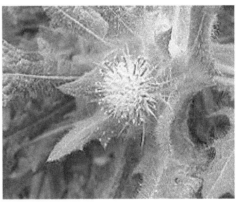

Cnicus benedictus (Rigeria
nyagutwa)

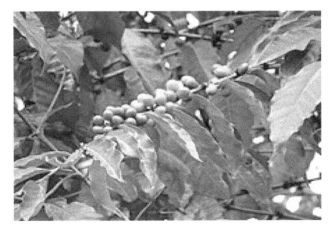

Coffea Arabica (Ekagwa)

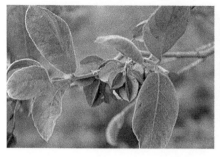

Combretum molle (Kamukira)

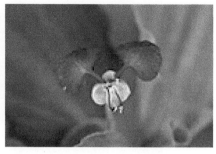

Commelina benghalensis (Rikongiro)

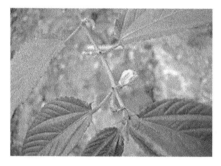

Corchorus olitorius (Omotere)

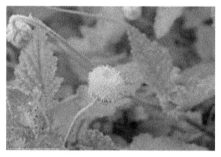

Crassocephalum vitellinum (Entamame)

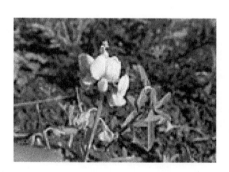

Crotalaria retusa L.

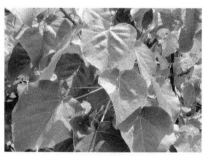

Croton macrostachyus (Omosocho)

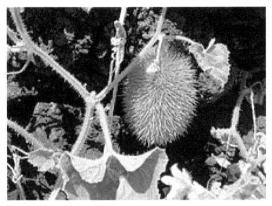

Cucumis disaceus Spach. (Obuya)

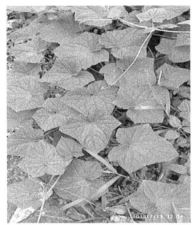

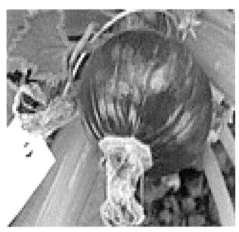

Cucumis prophetarum
(Omwatekania)

Cucurbita maxima (Omwongo)

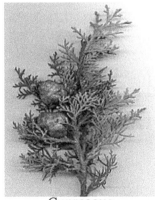

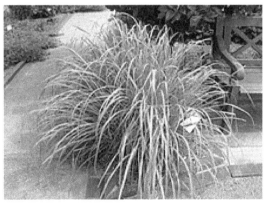

Cupressus
sempervivens
(Ebakora/Ekerobo)

Cymbopogon citratus (Obonyansi
bw'echae)

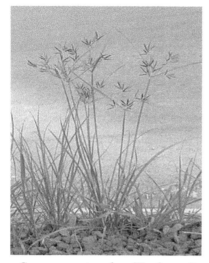

Cyperus rotundus (Endwani)

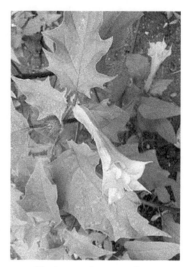

Datura stramonium
(Ekeroro)

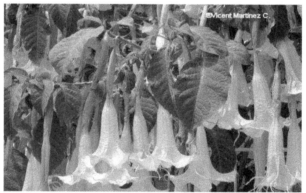

Datura arborea L (Ekeroria)

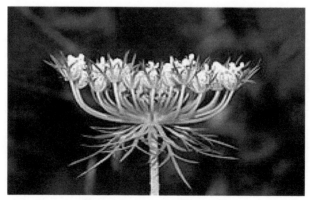

Daucus carota (Ekarati)

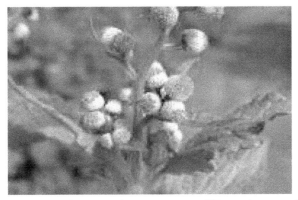

Dichrocephala integrifolia O. Kuntze (Ekeng'enta mbori)

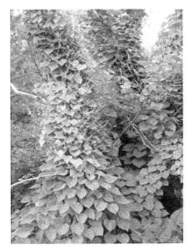

Dioscorea minutiflora
(Chinduma)

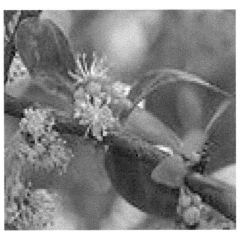

Dovyalis abyssinica
(Omokorogonywa)

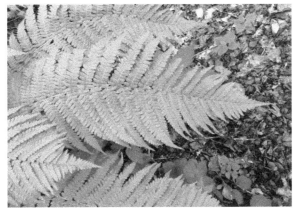

Dryopteris filix-mas (Eengwe)

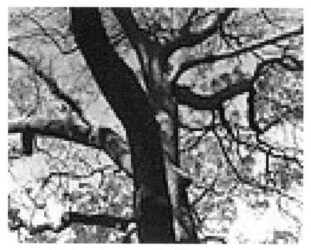

Ekebergia capensis (Omonyamari)

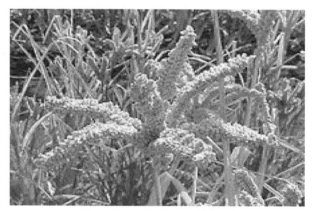

Eleusine coracana (Obori)

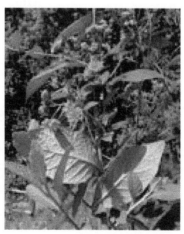

Erlangea marginata (Omonyaiboba)

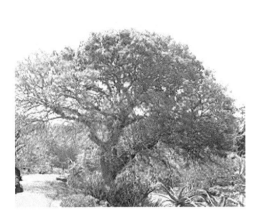

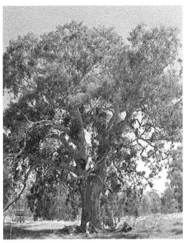

Erythrina abyssinica (Omotembe)

Eucalyptus camaldulensis
(Omoringamu omokong'u)

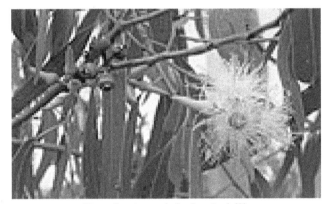

Eucalyptus globules Labill.
(Omoringamu bw'amache)

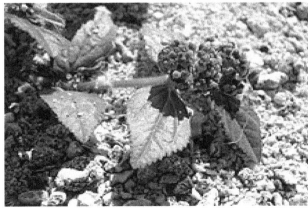

Euphorbia hirta L. (Obwaranse)

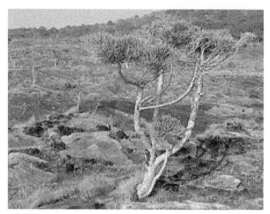

Euphorbia tirucalli L. (Ekerachwoki)

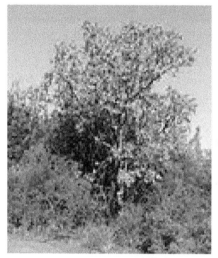

Fauera rochetiana (Omosasa)

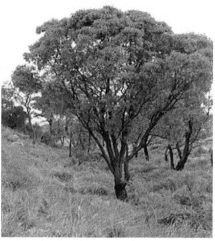

Faurea saligna (Omosasa omwegaroi)

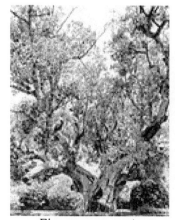

Ficus exasperate (*Omosenia*/Risenia)

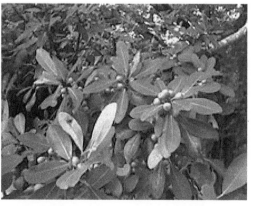

Ficus natalensis (Omogumo)

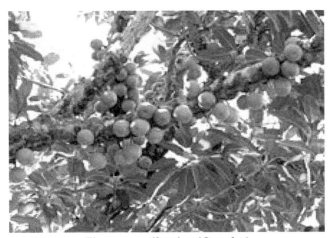

Ficus sansibarica (Omoko)

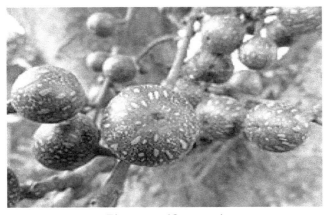

Ficus sur (Omoraa)

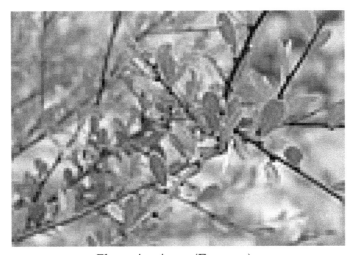

Flueggia virosa (Esarara)

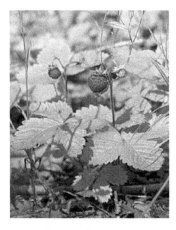

Fragaria vesca
(Chinkenene)

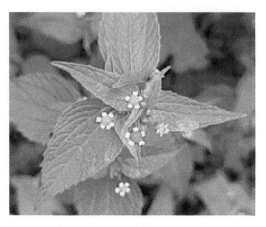

Galinsoga parviflora (Omenta)

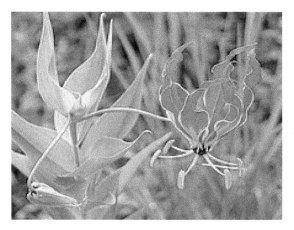

Gloriosa superba (Omorero bwenyang'au)

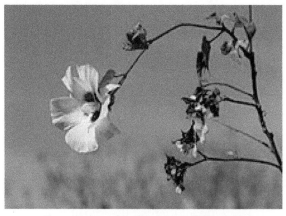

Gossypium barbadense (Ebamba)

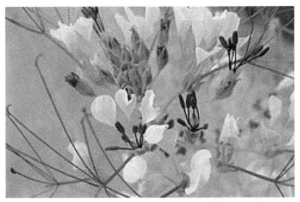

Gynandropsis gynandra (Chinsaga)

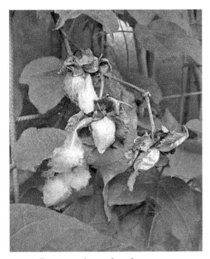

Gossypium herbaceum
(Ebamba)

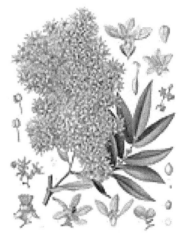

Hagennia abyssinica
(Omokunakuna)

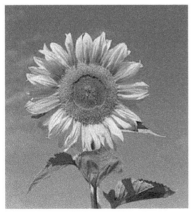

Helianthus annus (Riuga
ri'omogaso)

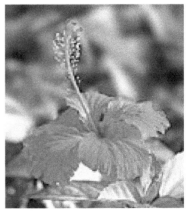

Hibiscus fuscus
(Egesiringi)

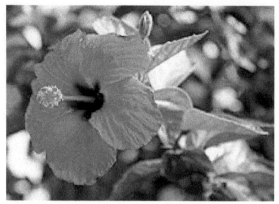

Hibiscus rosa-sinensis (Egesiringi ekiegarori)

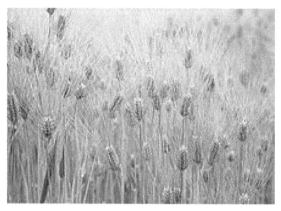

Hordeum vulgare (Engano)

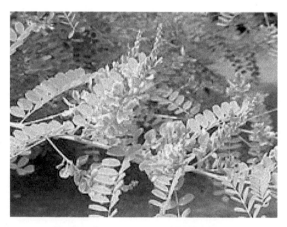

Indigofera arrecta (Omocheo)

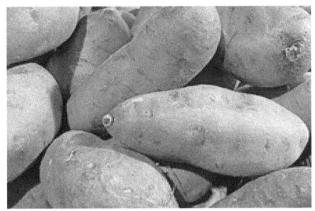

Ipomoea batatas (Amanyabwari)

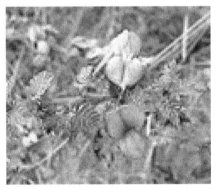

Kotschya africana (Omosing'oro)

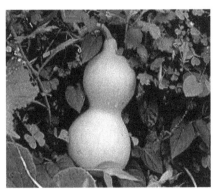

Lagenaria siceraria (Ekerandi)

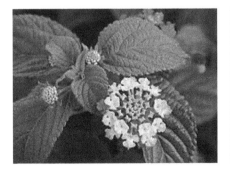

Lantana camara (Obori bw'enyoni)

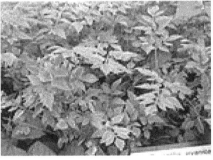

Lappia javanica (Omonyinkwa)

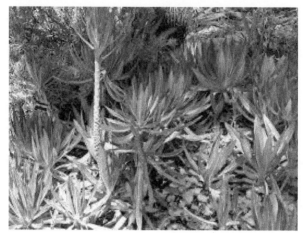

Lobelia gibberoa Hemsl (Omomoa/Etumbato enyegarori)

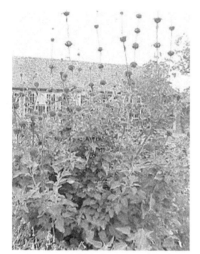

Leonotis nepetifolia (Risibi)

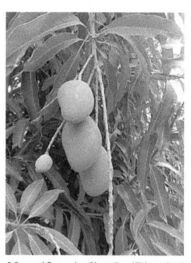

Mangifera indica L. (Riembe)

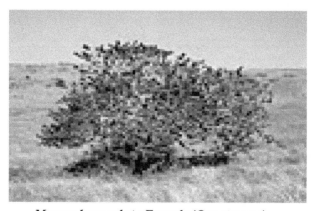

Maesa lanceolate Forssk (Omoterere)

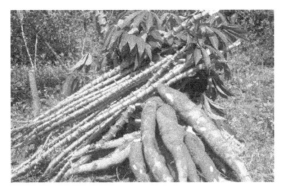

Manihot esculentum Crantz. (Omwogo)

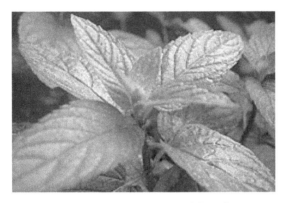

Mentha piperita L. (Mitisosi)

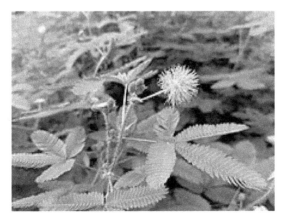

Mimosa pudica (L.) Del. (Ekiebundi)

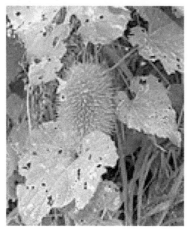

Mormodica foetida Schumach
(Egwagwa)

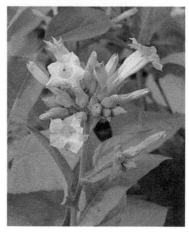

Nicotiana tabacum L.
(Etumbato)

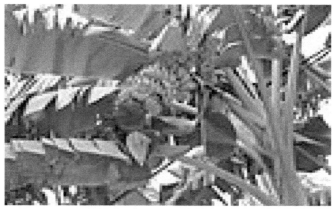

Musa paradisiaca subsp *sapientum* Kuntze (Ritoke)

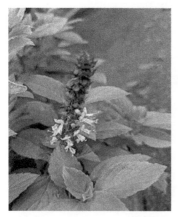

Ocimum kilimandscharicum
Guerke (Omote oitimo)

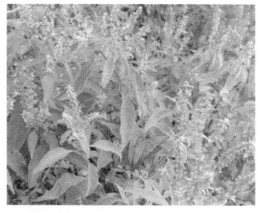

Ocimum suave Willd. (Omonyinkwa)

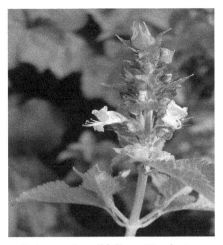

Ocimum lamiifolium Hochst ex Benth. (Esurancha)

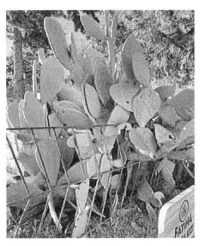

Opuntia ficus- indica (L.) Miller (exotic) (Omote bwa' amakengo)

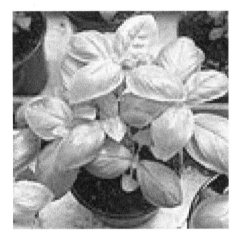

Ocinum basilicum L. (Ribuko)

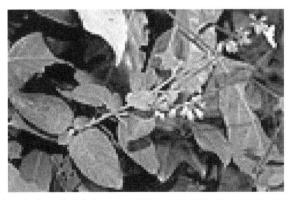

Orthosiphon hildebrandtii Benth. (Ekebungabaiseke)

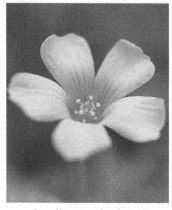

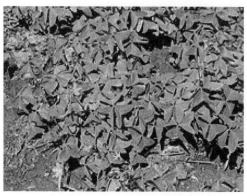

Oxalis corniculata L.
(Enyonyo enene)

Oxalis latifolia Kunth (Enyonyo)

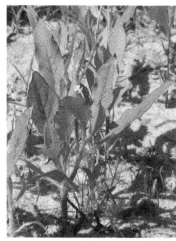

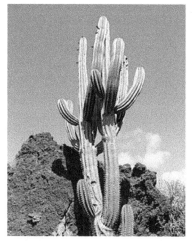

Oxygonum sinuatum (Hochst &
Steud ex. Meisn) (Omonyantira
omwegarori)

Pachycereus pectin-aboriginum L
(Engoto)

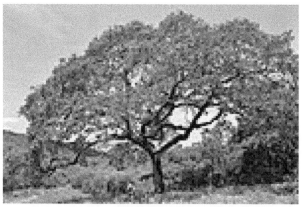

Parinari curatellifolia Benth (Omoraa)

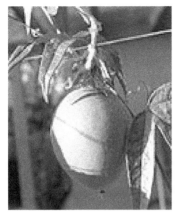

Passiflora incamata L.
(Ritindogoro (Ritunda
nyakoranda)

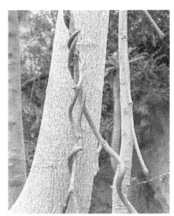

Pentarrhinum insipidium L.
(Ogoto kw'embeba)

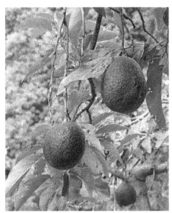

Persea gratissima (L.)
Gaertn. (Avocado)

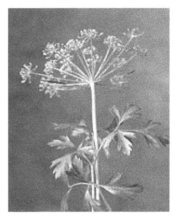

Petroselimum crispum (Mill)
Nyman. (Endania)

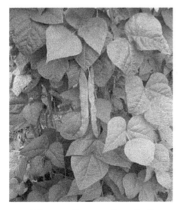

Phaseolus vulgaris L.
(Ching'ende)

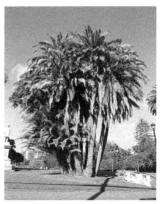

Phoenix reclinata Jacq.
(Rikendo)

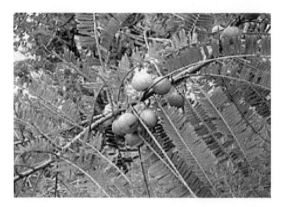

Phyllanthus avalifolius Forssk. (Omonyanaigo)

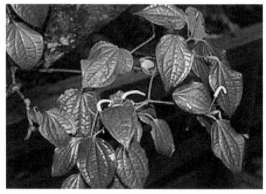

Piper capense L. (Ekenyanengo)

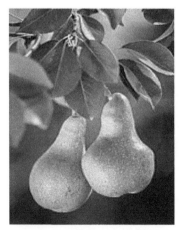

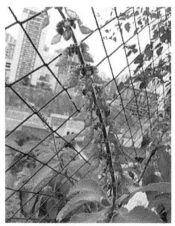

Pirus malus L. (exotic)
(Riembe)

Plectranthus barbatus
L'He'rit. (Omoroka)

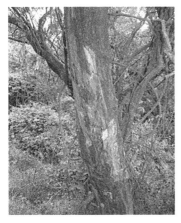

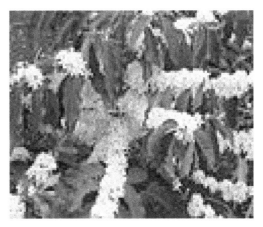

Prunus africana (Hook. f.) Kalkm. (Ekeburabura)

Psiada arabica Jacq (Omosune omonyerere)

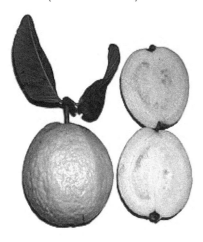

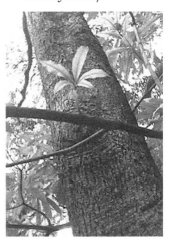

Psidium guajava L. (exotic) (Ripera)

Rauvolfia caffra Sond. (Omomure)

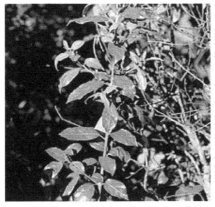

Rhamnus prinoides L' He'rit (Omong'ura)

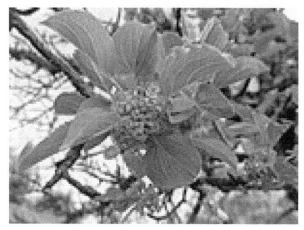

Rhamnus staddo A. Rich. (Omonyanengo)

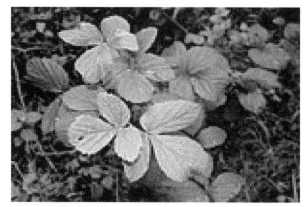

Rhoicissus tridentate (Omonyambeche/Egesanga)

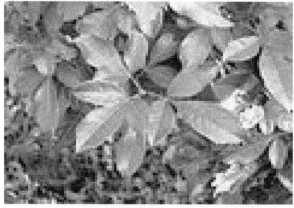

Rhus vulgaris Meikle (Obosangora)

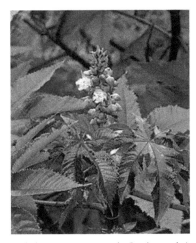
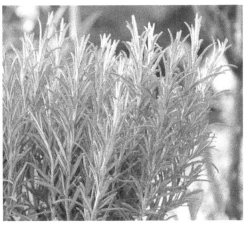

Ricinus communis L. (exotic) (Omobono)

Rosmarinus officinalis L. (Erosimeri)

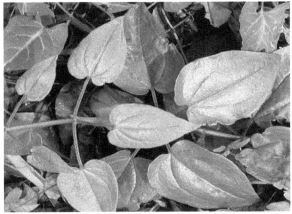

Rubia cordifolia L. (Eng'urang'uria)

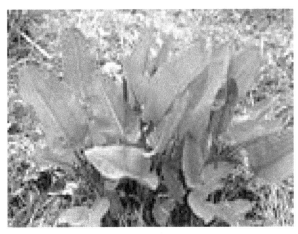

Rumex usambarensis Dammer. (Omonyantira)

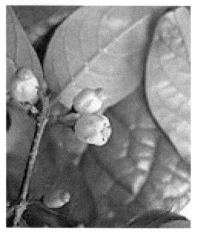

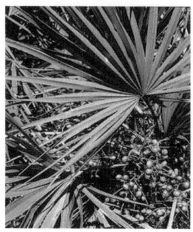

Rytigynia acuminatissima (K. Schum) Robyns (Omonyiinga)

Serenoa repens (Bartram) Small. (Rikendo riegarori)

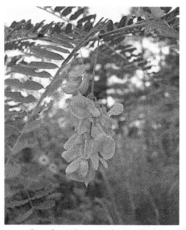

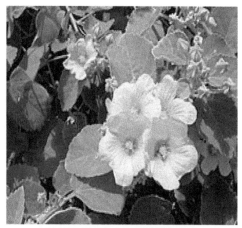

Sesbania sesban (L.) Merrill var. nubica Chiov. (Omosabisabi)

Sida tenuicarpa Vollesen. (Ekeburanchogu)

Sida cordifolia L. (Ekerundu)

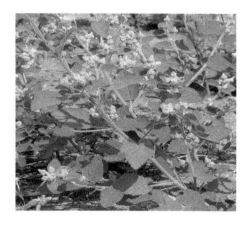

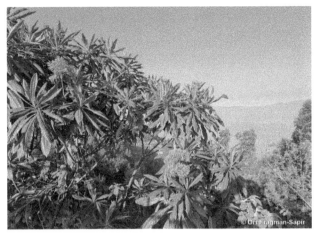

Solanecio mannii (Hook. f.) C. Jeffrey (Omotagara)

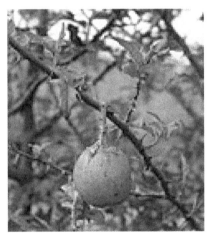

Solanum acueastrum Dunal (Omotobo)

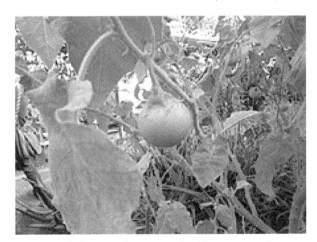

Solanum incanum L. (Omoratora)

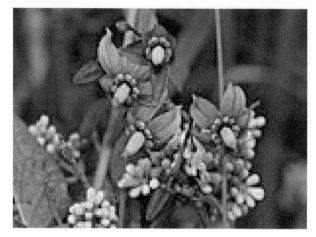

Solanum mauense Bitter. (Engeng'encha)

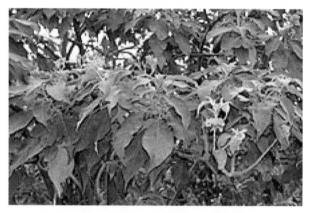

Solanum mauritianum Scop. (Omonsarigo)

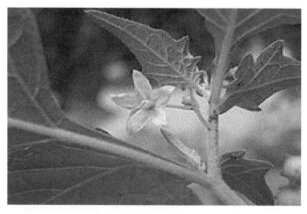

Solanum nigrum L. (Rinagu)

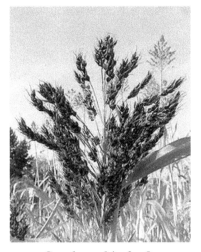

Sorghum bicolor L.
(*Amaemba*)

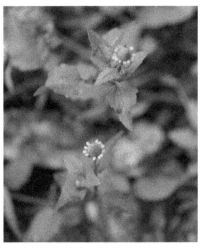

Spilanthes mauritiana (A. Rich)
DC. (Ekenyunyunta monwa)

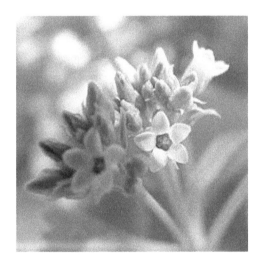

*Tabernaemontana
stapfiana* Britten
(Omobondo)

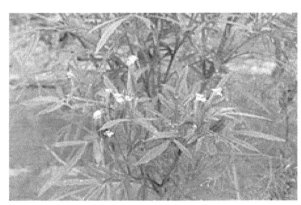

Tagetes minuta L.
(Omotiokia)

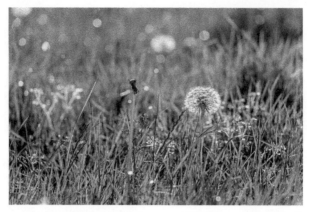

Taraxacum officinale Weber ex. Wiggers (Etandalioni)

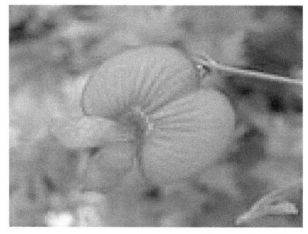

Tephrosia nana Kotschy & Schweinf. (Omochegechege)

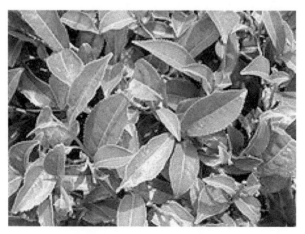

Thea sinensis L. (Echae)

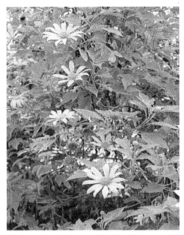

Tithonia diversifolia (Hemsl.)
Gray (exotic). (Riuga riroro)

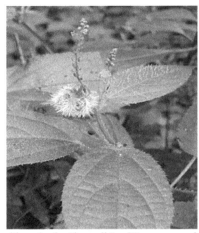

Tragia bethamii L. (Enyangeni
/Enyanduri)

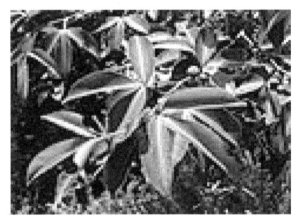

Toddalia asiastica (L.) Lam. (Ekenagwa ekiagarori)

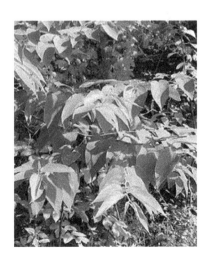

Trema orientalis (L). Bl.
(Omonyia)

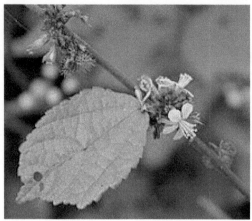

Triumfetta branchyceras K. Schum. (Ekemiso)

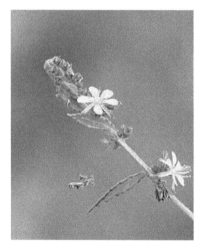

Triumfetta rhomboidea Jacq.
(Omomiso)

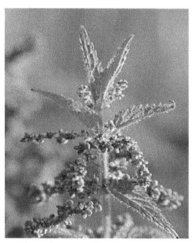

Urtica dioica L. (Rise)

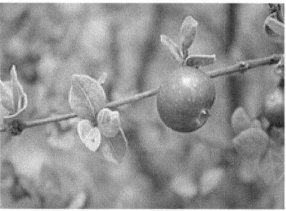

Vangueria apiculata K. Schum. (Omokomoni)

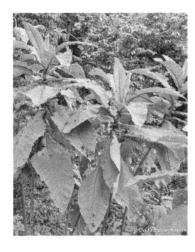

Vernonia auriculifera Hiern.
(Omosabakwa)

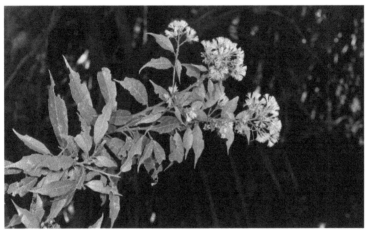

Vernonia amygdalina Del. (Omonyamosuto/Omorororia)

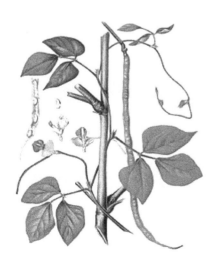

Vigna subterranean L.
(Chinchugu)

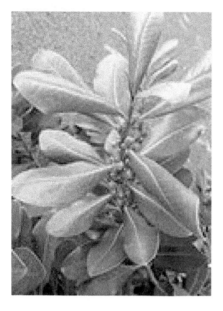 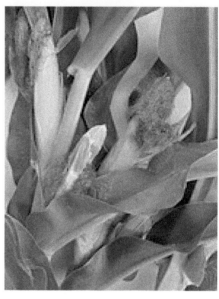

Warburgia ugandensis Sprague
(Esoko/Omonyakige)

Zea mays L. (Ebando/Egetuma)

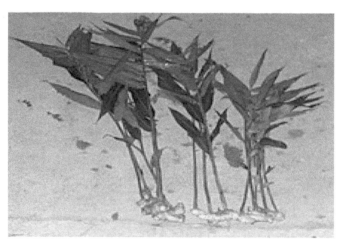

Zingiber officinale Roscoe (Entangausi)

Indices

Names of Plants in EkeGusii

E

Earare 77, 187

Ebakora 52, 191

Ebamba 62, 63, 198, 199

Ebando 57, 220

Echae 81, 216

Eengwe 39, 193

Egesanga 84, 210

Egesiringi 63, 199

Egesiringi ekiegarori 63, 200

Egetuma 57, 220

Egetunguo 61, 183

Egetunguo saumu 61, 183

Egwagwa 52, 204

Ekabichi nyamato 53, 186

Ekagwa 75, 189

Ekarati 81, 192

Ekebungabaiseke 60, 205

Ekeburabura 75, 209

Ekeburanchogu 64, 212

Ekemiso 80, 218

Ekemogamogia 46, 186

Ekenagwa 40, 77, 186, 187, 217

Ekenagwa ekiagarori 77, 217

Ekeng'enta mbori 47, 193

Ekenyambi 56, 182

Ekenyanengo 72, 208

Ekenyunyunta monwa 49, 215

Ekerachwoki 54, 196

Ekerandi 52, 201

Ekerobo 52, 62, 184, 191

Ekeroria 78, 192

Ekeroro 78, 192

Ekerundu 63, 212

Ekiebundi 66, 203

Emete y'amaiso 45, 183

Emoti 56, 184

Endania 82, 207

Enderema 39, 185

Endwani 53, 192

Engano 57, 200

Engeng'encha 79, 214

Eng'urang'uria 75, 211

Entamame 47, 190

Entangausi 84, 220

Enyanduri 56, 217

Enyangeni 56, 217

Enyasore 43, 187

Enyonyo 69, 206

Enyonyo enene 68, 206

Erosimeri 60, 211

Esarara 37, 55, 182, 197

Esoko 42, 220

Esurancha 59, 205

Etandalioni 50, 216

Etumbato 78, 204

Etumbato enyegarori 42, 202

Eyesura 65, 182

K

Kamukira 44, 190

M

Mitisosi 58, 203

O

Oboba 36, 182

Obonyansi bw'echae 57, 191

Obori 57, 194

Obori bw'enyoni 83, 201

Obosangora 38, 210

Names of Diseases in English

About the Author

William Gisesa was born at Botana in Nyamira County, located in the Gusii Highlands of South Western Kenya. He has a First Class Honours degree in Education (Botany and Zoology) from the University of Nairobi, a Masters (M.Sc.) degree in Plant Physiology and Biochemistry and a Doctor of Philosophy (PhD) in Ethnopharmacology from Kenyatta University.

Dr. Gisesa's main research interest is in Ethnopharmacology - the cross-cultural study of plants, animals and fungi or other naturally occurring resources used as medicines by ethnic and cultural groups. The main focus of the field has been on discovering drugs based on the therapeutic use of plants by indigenous people. Beyond the medical impact such studies reveal the importance of cultural and biological diversity and help with the conservation of cultural heritage.

The author is also interested in the processing of natural products in these categories: **1. Nutraceuticals,** e.g. value-added traditional foods, food flavourings, nutraceuticals, high energy food drinks, etc.; **2. Phytomedicines/ Phytopharmaceuticals,** e.g., Antimicrobials, Immune boosters, Anti-inflammatories, Pain killers, Laxatives, etc.; **3**. **Ethnoveterinary Products,** e.g., Acaricides, Dewormers, Food Supplements, Cattle Licking Blocks, etc.; **4**. **Body Care Products**, e.g., Herbal Soaps, Lotions, Perfumes, Shampoos, Mouth Washes, Toothpastes, etc.; **5**. **Household Care Products**, e.g., Detergents, Antiseptics, etc.; and **6**. **Organic Farm Inputs**, e.g., Biofertilizers, Biopesticides, etc. from biological resources.

He has published widely in scholarly journals including *Journal of Plant Sciences, Journal of Ethnomedicine, Journal of Ethnopharmacology*. He is co-author of *Gusii Proverbs in Contextual Usage* (in Press*)*. Currently, he is the Principal Researcher at The Global Institute of Traditional Medicine and Biotechnology.